# Health Impacts of Waste Management Policies

Environmental Science and Technology Library

VOLUME 16

*The titles published in this series are listed at the end of this volume.*

# Health Impacts of Waste Management Policies

Proceedings of the Seminar
'Health Impacts of Waste Management Policies',
Hippocrates Foundation, Kos, Greece, 12-14 November 1998

Edited by

P. Nicolopoulou-Stamati
*Department of Pathology,*
*Medical School,*
*National and Capodistrian University of Athens,*
*Athens, Greece*

L. Hens
*Human Ecology Department,*
*Vrije Universiteit Brussel,*
*Brussels, Belgium*

and

C.V. Howard
*Fetal and Infant Toxico-Pathology,*
*University of Liverpool,*
*Liverpool, England, United Kingdom*

KLUWER ACADEMIC PUBLISHERS
DORDRECHT / BOSTON / LONDON

A C.I.P. Catalogue record for this book is available from the Library of Congress.



ISBN 0-7923-6362-0

---

Published by Kluwer Academic Publishers,
P.O. Box 17, 3300 AA Dordrecht, The Netherlands.

Sold and distributed in North, Central and South America
by Kluwer Academic Publishers,
101 Philip Drive, Norwell, MA 02061, U.S.A.

In all other countries, sold and distributed
by Kluwer Academic Publishers,
P.O. Box 322, 3300 AH Dordrecht, The Netherlands.

Cover picture: Evening view from Weston Village, Runcorn, UK, over the ICI Castner-Kellner/Rocksavage site on the River Mersey estuary.

Desktop publishing by Glenn Ronsse

**Editorial Statement**

It is the policy of ASPIS to encourage the full spectrum of opinion to be represented at its meetings. Therefore it should not be assumed that the publication of a paper in this volume implies that the Editorial Board are fully in agreement with the contents, though we have tried to ensure that contributions are factually correct. Where, in our opinion, there is scope for ambiguity we have added footnotes to the text, where appropriate.

*Printed on acid-free paper*



Printed in the Netherlands.

# TABLE OF CONTENTS

# PREFACE AND ACKNOWLEDGEMENTS

The environmental health effects of waste management options such as waste deposition and incineration generate growing concern in society as a whole, and in a wide array of target groups in environmental management in particular. The latter include researchers, policy makers, journalists, NGO, lawyers, and medical professionals.

This book overviews the state of the art information at two levels:
a. the environmental health effects of waste management;
b. the interface with waste treatment policy.

The information mainly deals with household waste, although selected references to industrial waste are provided. This means that specific industrial waste streams, eventually with important health impacts, as nuclear waste, are not included.

The information contained in this book reveals that:
a. health risks are associated with waste disposal, incineration, related thermal treatment, and recycling;
b. many pollutants are associated with waste management practices, but specific attention is paid to halogenated hydrocarbons and particulates;
c. the risks concern mainly cancer, embryonic and fetal development, neurological and behavioural changes, immunological and reproductive effects;
d. although policy options in Europe and the US are not based upon health priorities, the prevailing hierarchy which is used in waste management (prevention - re-use - recycling - thermal decomposition - deposition) does not conflict with health data.

This book is based upon the proceedings of a workshop held in Kos, from November 12th - 14th, 1999. The workshop was organised in the framework of the ASPIS project.

This project aims at raising awareness on the most important environmental health issues. To this aim it gathers experts in different disciplines to exchange ideas on new policy tools for environmental education.

The editors of this book wish to thank the EU, the Greek Ministry of the Aegean Sea and the Greek Ministry of the Environment for their support. We wish also to thank the Municipality of Kos and the people who assisted in the organisation of the seminar.

The help of Glenn Ronsse, who bore the burden of the organisation, the editing and the desktop publishing of this book, and Mike Robbs and Craig Morrison who were in charge of the language review, is most sincerely appreciated.

The realisation of the ASPIS project involves a large number of people including students and university staff from the Department of Pathology, Medical School, University of Athens, the Department of Human Ecology, Free University Brussels (VUB) and the Department of Fetal & Infant Toxico-Pathology, University of Liverpool. To all of them we owe our most sincere appreciation.

| Polyxeni Nicolopoulou-Stamati | Luc Hens | Vyvyan C. Howard |
|---|---|---|
| Medical School | Human Ecology | Fetal & Infant Pathology |
| University of Athens | Department | Department |
| ASPIS Project Co-ordinator | Vrije Universiteit Brussel | University of Liverpool |

# LIST OF CONTRIBUTORS

P. DE BOER
*Neonatology Department*
*Emma Children's Hospital*
*Academic Medical Centre*
*University of Amsterdam*
*PO Box 22660*
*1100 DD Amsterdam*
*THE NETHERLANDS*

C. DONTAS
*Ministry of Environmental Housing*
*Planning and Public Works*
*Parnasidos 57*
*Chalandri*
*15321 Athens*
*GREECE*

L. HENS
*Vrije Universiteit Brussel*
*Human Ecology Department*
*Laarbeeklaan 103*
*B-1090 Brussel*
*BELGIUM*

C.V. HOWARD
*University of Liverpool*
*Fetal & Infant Toxico-Pathology*
*P.O. Box 147*
*L69 7ZA Liverpool*
*UNITED KINGDOM*

G. KAMIZOULIS
*WHO/EURO Project Office*
*Mediterranean Action Plan*
*Vassileos Konstantinou 48*
*11635 Athens*
*GREECE*

J.G. KOPPE
*Neonatology Department*
*Emma Children's Hospital*
*Academic Medical Centre*
*University of Amsterdam*
*PO Box 22660*
*1100 DD Amsterdam*
*THE NETHERLANDS*

J. LAFERE
*Vrije Universiteit Brussel*
*Human Ecology Department*
*Laarbeeklaan 103*
*B-1090 Brussel*
*BELGIUM*

R.L. LINDBAUER
*AE Energietechnik*
*P.O.B. 1004*
*A-8021 Graz*
*AUSTRIA*

O. LINHER
*European Commission, DG III*
*Wetstraat 200*
*B-1049 Brussels*
*BELGIUM*

P. NICOLOPOULOU-STAMATI
*National and Capodistrian University of Athens*
*Medical School, Department of Pathology*
*75, Micres Ajias, GOYDI*
*11527 Athens*
*GREECE*

M. PARKES
*University of Otago*
*Wellington School of Medicine*
*Ecology & Health Research Centre*
*PO Box 7343*
*Wellington*
*NEW ZEALAND*

P. RUSHBROOK
*Regional Advisor, Waste Management*
*WHO Rome Operational Division*
*Via Francesco Crispi 10*
*00187 Rome*
*ITALY*

D. SOTIROPOULOS-VARDAKA
*European Environmental Bureau*
*Bld. de Waterloo 34*
*B-1000 Brussels*
*BELGIUM*

G. STAATS DE YANES
*WHO-Centre*
*Tierärztlichen Hochschule Hannover*
*Bünteweg 2*
*D-30559 Hannover*
*GERMANY*

G.A. STAM
*Neonatology Department*
*Emma Children's Hospital*
*Academic Medical Centre*
*University of Amsterdam*
*PO Box 22660*
*1100 DD Amsterdam*
*THE NETHERLANDS*

C. STEENWEGEN
*AMINAL*
*Graaf De Ferraris Bldg. 3th floor*
*Emiel Jacqmainlaan 156 bus 8*
*B-1000 Brussels*
*BELGIUM*

G. TEN TUSSCHER
*Neonatology Department*
*Emma Children's Hospital*
*Academic Medical Centre*
*University of Amsterdam*
*PO Box 22660*
*1100 DD Amsterdam*
*THE NETHERLANDS*

G. VALAORAS
*University of La Verne*
*Athens Campus*
*PO Box 51105*
*14510 Kifissia*
*GREECE*

L. VAN GRIMBERGEN
*Flemish Public Waste Agency*
*(Openbare Vlaamse*
*Afvalstoffenmaatschappij)*
*Kan. de Deckerstraat 22-26*
*B-2800 Mechelen*
*BELGIUM*

N. VAN LAREBEKE
*Department of Radiotherapy, Nuclear*
*Medicine and Experimental Cancerology*
*University of Gent*
*De Pintelaan 185*
*B-9000 Gent*
*BELGIUM*

# LIST OF FIGURES

# LIST OF TABLES

# LIST OF BOXES

# INTRODUCTORY CHAPTER: AWARENESS OF THE HEALTH IMPACTS OF WASTE MANAGEMENT

*Introduction to and Overview of the Proceedings of the Seminar*

*'Health Impacts of Waste Management Policies'*

*Hippocrates Foundation, Kos, Greece, 12-14 November, 1998*

P. NICOLOPOULOU-STAMATI[1]
C.V. HOWARD[2]
M. PARKES[3]
L. HENS[4]
*[1]National and Capodistrian University of Athens*
*Medical School, Department of Pathology*
*75, Micres Ajias, GOYDI*
*11527 Athens, GREECE*
*[2]University of Liverpool*
*Fetal & Infant Toxico-Pathology*
*P.O. Box 147*
*L69 7ZA Liverpool, UNITED KINGDOM*
*[3]University of Otago*
*Wellington School of Medicine*
*Ecology & Health Research Centre*
*PO Box 7343*
*Wellington, NEW ZEALAND*
*[4]Vrije Universiteit Brussel*
*Human Ecology Department*
*Laarbeeklaan 103*
*B-1090 Brussels, BELGIUM*



*P. Nicolopoulou-Stamati et al. (eds.), Health Impacts of Waste Management Policies,* 1–25.

**Summary**

This chapter introduces key themes from the book, reflecting the topics of the 'Awareness of the Health Impacts of Waste Management Policies' Seminar, in Kos, Greece, November, 1998. The waste management and health scene is introduced by an outline of concerns relating to persistent organic pollutants, as well as through perspectives from Less Developed Countries and from industry. An overview of policy lines for waste management includes an assessment of recent proposals by the European Commission, as well as selected examples from European countries and the USA. Descriptions of developments in research, tools and conceptual approaches for waste management and health issues are provided. Research into health effects of dioxins and PCBs is outlined, as are reviews of technological options for waste management, proposed developments in health impact assessment, environmental taxes as a waste management tool, and integrated regional waste management approaches. A series of case studies provide real-world examples of research and policy development including a review of the effects of waste management on wildlife and domestic animals. In conclusion, important crossover themes and challenges are outlined. Topical issues include differences between technological capacity and actual performance, burden of proof and the precautionary principle, hazard versus risk assessment, and societal dimensions of awareness and attitudes. Time-lag, intergenerational effects and the introduction of the chemical hygiene concept are highlighted as important considerations, as well as the general need for prioritisation of the child and infant in all regulatory procedures. Such themes highlight the need for both scientific and policy advance in response to the links between waste management and public health.

## 1. Introduction

ASPIS, the Greek word for a shield, is also the acronym for **A**wareness **S**trategies for **P**ollution from **I**ndu**S**tries, a project funded under DG 11 and later under DG 16 of the EU. Its main aim has been to raise awareness - amongst politicians, lawyers, medical practitioners, regulators, journalists and other decision-makers - of global pollution and environmental health problems. This has been achieved firstly by organising a series of meetings in Belgium, Greece and the UK; at which the subjects discussed included pesticides, fresh and recreational water, halogenated pollutants and xenoestrogens. Secondly, ASPIS has disseminated information on aspects of pollution which has been widely distributed. The organisers of ASPIS firmly believe that it is only by the process of raising awareness amongst policy-makers about the serious environmental pollution problems that exist and need to be addressed, that action to reverse some of the more pressing matters will come about.

This seminar was arranged as part of a series, with the specific aim of bringing together various groups of technical experts and decision-makers in a setting inducive to frank and fair exchange of ideas and information concerning health impacts of the manner in which society deals with its waste problems. The seminar consisted of formal presentations by the participants, and extended debating and discussion periods. This volume summarises the findings.

The structure of the contents mirrors the order in which the topics were presented and discussed in Kos. This follows a logical progression:

The session on waste management and the health scene highlighted the state of knowledge of the adverse health effects of pollutants produced by the incineration and land filling of waste, as measured by toxicological and epidemiological research. With respect to dioxin-like substances, it has become clear that a proportion of the population in developed countries already has a body burden which is high enough to be causing measurable effects in the following generations. Health effects associated with living in the vicinity of landfill sites were emphasised.

The health and waste management policies employed in a number of industrialised countries, including Austria, Belgium, Greece, the UK and the USA, were analysed.

There followed a series of case studies addressing different aspects of waste management and health. These presentations were amongst the most informative for the decision-makers among the delegates. Topics addressed included: the measurable health effects of waste incineration on children. Two presentations outlined the incidence of congenital malformations in the vicinity of incineration sites. Finally an appraisal of the impact of waste policy on the contamination of food of animal origin emphasised the vulnerability of humankind to the effects of bio-concentration and bio-magnification up the food web. This paper has proven, with hindsight, to be somewhat prescient in the light of the recent Brazilian citrus pulp and Belgian dioxin food scandals, which have been uncovered since this volume was compiled.

This introductory chapter gives an overview of the papers which were presented at the conference and published as full papers in these proceedings. The conclusions focus on the main lines of thought expressed during the conference. As such they provide basic rules of thumb on health and waste management.

## 2. Waste Management and the Health Scene

Vyvyan Howard's keynote contribution entitled **'Persistent Organic Chemical Pollution'** introduces the increasing concern over the nature and extent of a variety of health effects relating to Waste Management.

The example of organochlorine compounds is used to demonstrate growing awareness of health impacts of waste which extend beyond direct acute health effects, and include chronic and less direct effects with the capacity for long-term health impact, including that of the next generation. Organochlorines are notable for being almost entirely anthropogenic products, resulting from the combination of the industrial by-product of chlorine with hydrocarbons in other industrial processes such chemical and pesticide manufacturing, pulp and paper bleaching, or incineration. Whether produced as an unwanted product or by-product in the waste stream, organochlorines are a substance alien to vertebrate biochemistry. As such they exhibit important properties, impacting human health, as listed below:

i) they are extremely *stable and persistent* compounds;
ii) their lipophilic nature means they *bio-accumulate*;
iii) many are *toxic* with *bioactivity* occurring at low levels (similar to that which gives bioactivity to hormones). The toxicity of this kind of waste is associated with the triad of non-cancer effects of *immunosuppression*, *hormone disruption*, and *neurodevelopmental deficit*.

Awareness of these concepts enables understanding of why organochlorines transfer up the food chain to humans through animal fat, as well as from mothers to the next generation via the placenta and breast milk. The developing foetus is the most sensitive part of the human life cycle, and is particularly prone to the toxicity of lipophilic substances due their high exposure per unit body weight and their low body fat stores.

Dioxins provide an example of one of the most widely studied and best understood groups of organochlorines, which have been shown by US EPA research to be mostly derived from incinerated medical and municipal waste. Although technology has improved, it is important to note that the difference between actual and potential technological capacity makes technological solutions to the organochlorine problem risky in the context of both landfills and incineration. This is especially due to the fact that although organochlorines may be transformed to gas, particulates or ash, the precursors or toxic substances will persist in some form in the environment with potential health effects.

The concept of *existing body burden* is proposed as important in increasing the awareness of the health impact of waste. Current methods to determine safe levels of waste substances are dangerously limited if they do not take into account the known and existing high body burden of substances such as organochlorines. Body burden should be recognised as especially important due to chronic exposure and bio-accumulation, as well as in relation to the multiple compounds with potential health impacts present in waste.

Current methods for estimating health effects are generally limited to single substances and do not take into account the potential accumulative and synergistic effects of exposure to, and body burden of, complex mixtures. Sciences such as toxicology and epidemiology are already challenged by the health effects of single substances, and are faced with further limitations and uncertainties when dealing with complex mixtures. In acknowledging this, it is to be emphasised that the precautionary principle should be adopted for decision-making regarding health impacts of both the manufacture of products produced as well as their management as waste.

Philip Rushbrook contributes with a paper entitled **'The Challenge to Achieve Better Landfills Where Only Dumps are Achieved Now: An Anthology'**. A major theme here is the need to see the health effects of waste management within the larger context of public health challenges of the country under consideration. A variety of examples of this view are provided, drawing upon Mr. Rushbrook's own field experience in Eastern European countries where waste management does not have the same resources or options available as in more developed countries, and is not necessarily a public health priority.

It is noted that most available technological options for waste management are for non-organic and combustible rubbish. Incinerators in particular are not relevant for non-burnable waste, such as the municipal waste of high organic content characteristic of many less developed countries (LDCs). This determines why landfills are the only credible option for one hundred and seventy-five countries in the world, with the majority being open dumping.

In terms of health impact, Mr. Rushbrook reports data and figures relating to acute effects that result from direct exposure to those living near, working at or scavenging from landfills. In LDCs this is important in terms of increased gastro-intestinal, respiratory, eye infections/irritation, and general increase in morbidity and infant mortality. In more developed countries, Mr. Rushbrook concludes, waste management is relatively safe. The major attributable health impacts described are physical injuries to those working at waste disposal sites which, at a rate equivalent to that of construction workers, have little impact on the general public.

A global summary of the health effects of waste are ranked into four main categories.

i) direct physical harm;
ii) infective transmission of microbiological agents (re-emergence of malaria and rabies, rat-borne typhus and leptosporidiosis, and other bacterial and protozoal pathogens);
iii) chemical induced illness;
iv) reproductive interference.

In relation to reproductive interference, Mr. Rushbrook notes that there is a gradually increasing dossier of circumstantial evidence regarding birth defects, including a statistical relationship with landfills described in the EUROHAZCON study (Dolk *et al.*, 1998). However, since no definitive causal link has been demonstrated between Waste Management and birth defects, these findings are still viewed as inconclusive.

The global ranking list and the country variations are used to support the proposal that realistic standard-setting should take into account the priorities and capacity of the specific country. In this way standards can gradually increase as they have in developed countries, with initial priority being given to the health effects due to close proximity, then to standards to prevent direct environmental contamination, then finally to fine-tuning environmental health impact.

Using the example of Eastern Europe, Mr. Rushbrook reports that the main health concerns of the public were prioritised as: poor quality of air and drinking water; radiation levels; low housing standards; and food safety. Waste did not feature as a direct prioritised concern. This was interpreted as meaning that health effects of waste were not a public health priority or political issue and thus health concerns have little influence on waste management policy.

In particular it is emphasised that in LDCs waste management is a matter of choosing appropriate technology. Hi-tech equipment has limited relevance when set-up and maintenance costs are prohibitive. Even in urgent situations such as the recent stockpiling of expired medical supplies donated to Bosnia, poor understanding and prioritisation of health risks resulted in the only achievable solution being the cement-sealing of the medicines in barrels, despite possible incineration facilities.

The contribution by Otto Linher (EU DGIII) is entitled **'Waste Management: An Industrial Policy Point of View'**. Key concepts such as the EU waste management hierarchy and producer responsibility were discussed as well as EU legislation with an effect of reducing health impacts from waste management. The waste hierarchy gives preference to prevention, followed by recovery (including recycling and incineration with recovery) and final disposal. Advantages and limitations of this rule were discussed.

The fundamental objective of EU Waste Management Policy as outlined in the Waste Management Strategy is to achieve a *'high degree of environmental protection without distorting the functioning of the internal market with a view to promoting sustainable development'*. Within this framework the health impact of waste is referred to indirectly.

It needs to be noted that waste is one of the consequences of modern life which also has helped to produce the most healthy and long-living generation of mankind. This should, however, not hide the need to minimise waste production and the environmental impacts associated with waste treatment. The choice of waste management options is usually one of trade-offs, i.e. some health and environmental impacts are replaced by others. Re-use and recycling frequently helps to reduce such impacts but are in no way free from causing environmental pollution themselves.

More direct reference to the health effects of waste are made in a brief comparison of effects of incineration and landfills as key waste management options. Main health effects of landfill relate to the potential for groundwater contamination by leachate and the release of methane and toxic gases into the air (the latter e.g. by fires). As regards incinerator emissions, the issue of particulate matter emissions, partly through secondary formation from $NO_x$ and $SO_2$, seems to be the most serious as regards health impacts. Further pollutants that need to be addressed in emission limit values are heavy metals, dioxins and furans. The main problem with respect to environmental protection from waste is not so much the setting of standards for installation as their consequent implementation in practice.

## 3. National Policy Lines on Waste Management

This section starts with a contribution by Dioni Vardaka-Sotiropoulos from the umbrella organisation of the environmental organisations in Europe introducing **'The European Environmental Bureau on the European Commission's Proposal on Incineration of Waste'**. This provides some indication of the motivation behind and key alterations in the new directive, which included prioritising co-incineration of waste (incineration + energy production), updating of emission limit values for dioxins and furans to 0.1 $mg/m^3$, and the integration of latest technology. The EEB welcomed the change but emphasised need for emphasis further up the EEB preferred waste hierarchy including prevention, re-use, useful application (recycling), incineration and landfill.

The EEB response to the proposed changes demonstrates both environmental and health impact concerns. The EEB position prioritises obligatory co-incineration, integrated permitting, mandatory pre-treatment of waste, stricter emission values, and the promotion of a combined approach between Emission Limit Values (ELV) and Ambient Quality Objectives (AQO). As a measure of environmental state, AQOs may be considered a better proxy of human exposure and thus could be seen as more specific to determining and controlling for health impact.

The EEB also remained critical of the health implications of the 'damage-cost approach' used in the Cost-Benefit Analyses (CBA) in EU prioritisation. By focusing on mortality instead of morbidity, many chronic health effects and quality of life issues are not accounted for. Furthermore, the assumptions of CBA are not able to deal with chronic and synergistic health effects. For this reason, the EEB also advocates the application of the precautionary principle for waste management.

Four country presentations follow the EU's position. They include **'Household Waste Management' - in Flanders, Belgium** (L. Van Grimbergen) - **in Austria** (R.L. Lindbauer) - **in Greece** (C. Dontas) and **in the USA** (G. Valaoras).

In general the overviews of household waste management strategies did not reveal strong emphasis on the links between health impact and waste management, since in many cases health effects are considered as an implicit contribution to the need for waste management, but rarely specifically detailed.

In **Flanders, Belgium** the key objective of the waste management strategy is to protect human health and the environment, but few details are provided other than air emission levels for incinerators. Proposed developments are described in terms of new tools for waste management rather than new or increased health concerns.

The presentation of **Austria**'s Waste management strategies emphasises that *'the essential objective of all provisions relating to waste disposal is protection of human* *health and environment...'*. This paper is contributed by Mr. Ralf Lindbauer who acts as vice-chairman and is head of the waste management group of the European Committee of Environmental Technology Suppliers Associations. The focus is presented as the capacity of incinerators to act as a sink for toxic substances. This paper proposes a technological solution to the problem of miscellaneous toxins in the waste stream and ambient environment, supporting the phasing out of Austria's current landfills within the next 10 years. Key concepts include that of *waste* representing displaced products, *hazard* representing a potential danger from displaced products, and *risk* being the probability of this hazard happening. Incineration is presented as a safe, controlled way to reduce this risk. *Material flow analysis* is described as a tool to find out what substances are in the waste stream and in what way incinerators could act as a sink.

Mr. Constantin Dontas' contribution on **'Policy Options for Waste Management in Greece'** gives a comprehensive account of the Waste Management strategy currently being adopted in Greece. This provides a detailed account of the important considerations of locational variation between the major urban centres, the large fluctuations of waste in those islands with a tourist-based economy, and the specific requirements of rural and mountainous regions.

Health is not stated as an overt consideration when taking into account the background, available technology, budget, education and information availability of the different regions in order to develop a general hierarchy of waste management. This hierarchy is prioritised as follows:

a. recycling of 28.5 per cent of the waste stream;
b. composting plus anaerobic biogas production for the 47 per cent biodegradable waste;
c. sanitary landfills for the remaining 20 per cent.

Incineration is criticised not according to its health impact but simply because it is perceived as disadvantageous for Greece due to the high humidity of the waste stream and the concern regarding its incompatibility with the chosen prioritisation of recycling. The developing technologies of pyrolysis and gasification are both considered as possible future innovations, but are finally judged as too expensive and uncertain to be general solutions to the current problem.

Specific attention is given to the financing of the proposed Greek waste management strategy. First priority is given to establishing sanitary landfills to end current unsustainable practices, such as uncontrolled dumping, that have significant health and environmental impact. Another important priority is the rehabilitation of old dumping sites, and finally, investment into environmental justice considerations of new initiatives. This latter consideration recognises the need for consultation and planning to offset inequitable distribution of health and environmental impacts. A third way concerns composting. Special attention is given to industrial and hospital waste management. Although not providing details of specific health impacts, this prioritisation implicitly acknowledges the important health and quality of life impacts that result from waste management practices.

In general this paper suggests that a high level of integrated thinking, including health impact, has featured in the development of the proposed Greek Waste Management Strategy.

The presentation of the **USA** waste management strategy provides some detailed information regarding health effects in the forms of a report on recent epidemiological evidence regarding the health impact of landfills, with particular emphasis on the foetus (REHW, 1998). The release of municipal landfill gas and leachate to groundwater are referred to, the composition of which has been found to be the same as that produced at hazardous waste sites. Health effects reported included a fourfold increase in bladder cancer and leukaemia, and reports of raised incidence of several other cancers. Reference is made to low birthweight, and the small size of children as the most common effect of living near landfills, as well as recent studies showing an increase in birth defects.

Following this introduction to health effects of waste management, it is emphasised that although US waste management is basically dependant on individual states and municipalities, the US EPA makes federal decisions regarding health impact based on the procedure of *Risk Assessment.* An overview of the risk assessment paradigm is provided, emphasising its basis in science and methods for deriving a common measurement of health risk in order to allocate resources. The procedures for Hazard Identification, Dose-Response (toxicity) Assessment, Exposure Assessment and Risk Characterisation are outlined as methods used to quantify adverse effects of the substance, its probability, the extent of human exposure and the risks to public health. In addition problems with this method are referred to, including the difficult links between Risk Characterisation and Risk Management. Considerations include the perception of the risk of health impacts, and the limitations of dealing with multiple substances whose effects are simply added, rather than dealing with potential synergies.

A presentation was given in Kos on the UK position by Alan Watson. This is not reported in this volume but a resume of what was reported at the conference is given below.

The presentation regarding the United Kingdom noted that the generation of political action was largely health-based, with public interest groups having an important role in bringing environmental health issues into the political arena. The Environmental Agency is not in itself very health-focused, its main emphasis being a two-tiered system of planning and control. The general government strategy focused on individual and corporate responsibility to make sustainable choices.

In relation to the incineration versus landfill debate, currently the majority of UK waste is landfilled in continuation of historic precedent. This has raised increasing concern, especially highlighted by the EUROHAZCON study (Dolk *et al.*, 1998) and research findings showing that the incidence of the birth defect of gastroschisis near to a South Wales landfill is over twenty times higher than the national incidence. Meanwhile the incineration debate is heating up, with the key area being dioxin effects, but important issues of large scale contamination and body burden are not addressed. Recent Dutch, US and WHO data on the issue emphasise that a high level of care is needed. Breast-feeding remains of high concern with levels exceeding the UK norm by twenty times and the WHO norm by two hundred times.

## 4. Health Issues on Waste Management

Janna Koppe, a neonatologist from the University of Amsterdam opens this section of the proceedings focusing on health issues, with a presentation entitled **'Background Exposure to Dioxins and PCBs in Europe and the Resulting Health Effects'**. Awareness of the health impact of waste management is obviously the central aim of this paper, with a focus on dioxins as a toxic substance produced through waste incineration, and is especially important for the burgeoning population of Europe. The highest global levels of dioxin toxic equivalents (I-TEQs) in breast milk were shown to be found in the Netherlands, Belgium, Germany and the UK.

The starting point for presenting health impacts is with reference to adults. Clinical presentations include chloracne, hyperpigmentation, hirsutism, liver cirrhosis, polyneuropathies, tiredness and immunosuppression. Laboratory data include biochemically elevated levels of liver enzymes, raised prothrombin time, increased cholesterol and triglyceride levels.

Concern over health effects in young children is not related to ambient levels, since background levels are not high enough to produce symptoms. Instead the properties of dioxins in terms of their stability, bio-accumulation and lipophilicity facilitate understanding of how chronic bio-accumulation of dioxins in maternal fat-stores leads to toxic levels of TEQs in breast milk. Chronic sources of intake for mothers includes fish and other animal fats, for which there are no currently monitored standards in the Netherlands.

The core of this presentation is Janna Koppe's own research in the Netherlands (especially relating to disrupted Vitamin K and thyroid function) and the link between these findings and numerous other epidemiological studies around the world, where health effects in children have been associated with exposure to toxic incinerator emissions, including dioxin-like substances and furans. A brief summary of these findings is listed below.

- Toxic effects in infant and child as evidenced through *deranged thyroid regulation*, *decreased Vitamin K function*, and *deranged liver enzymes*.

- Vitamin K deficiency as evidenced in increased rates of a rare (1/100,000) form of infant haemorrhagic disease known as *late haemorrhagic disease* presented as intracranial bleeding at 1-3 months. Rates as high as 5/1000 are reported in Japan.
- *Developmental immunotoxicity* resulting in increased otitis and respiratory disease.
- *Impaired cognitive and motoric development* (hyperactivity and decreased IQ).
- *Skin abnormalities.*

The final message of Janna Koppe's presentation addresses the problem that 10 per cent of women in the Netherlands have been found to have a TEQ body burden that is greater than the level (19 ng TEQ) that is known to cause abnormalities in non-human primates. With the knowledge that breast feeding has many important health advantages for the infant, should Dutch woman still breastfeed? The suggestion from Dr Koppe is that breast feeding women should maintain their body fat and avoid losing weight in order to limit the circulating levels of dioxins.

Although this section does not analyse the possible health effects of all pollutants emitted by waste deposit sites and incinerators, it aims at addressing the main ones. In **'Particulate Aerosols, Incinerators and Health'** Vyvyan Howard starts from the finding that even the most modern waste incinerators emit aerosols of ultrafine particles which current filter technology does not abate. It has been shown that the inhalation of these ultrafine particles is associated with health effect such as blood coagulability and increased incidence of cardiovascular disease. The author also raises (unanswered) questions on the synergistic effects of these small particles with other pollutants such as heavy metals. Also the possible consequences of simultaneous exposure to different sources with similar pollutants such as vehicle emissions are addressed.

It cannot be excluded that these extra fine particulates ($PM_{<25}$) provide the most important health risk associated with modern incinerators. In view of the important scientific uncertainty, the paper concludes that there is an urgent need for research on the health impacts which might result from aerosols emitted by current incinerators. Moreover he advocates that the issue should be raised explicitly in future applications to licence waste incinerators.

The uncertainties and problems involved in estimating health effects from standards is a central introductory theme in the contribution entitled **'Health and Environmental Impact Assessment'** by Luc Hens. This presentation refers to the growing requirement for Health Impact Assessment (HIA) as part of Environmental Impact Assessment (EIA) of proposed projects. Decisions regarding waste management options such as incinerators or landfills require this form of assessment. This paper is therefore based on the specific and increasingly important scenario relating to awareness of health impact and how this can be more accurately predicted for proposed initiatives such as waste management developments.

The author refers to a study in Flanders assessing the methods used for the evaluation of human health in EIA. The common rationale is found to involve comparing predicted emission/immission levels of a substance with the standard or guideline relating to it. If the standards are not exceeded, the judgement is that there is no danger to health. This approach was criticised on two levels:

i) Environmental standards tell us very little about target organs, since it is very difficult to extrapolate an emission limit such as 0.1 ng/m$^3$ for dioxins to exposure and effects.
ii) Most standards in environmental laws tell us very little about health effects, since they are frequently based on Best Available Technology, rather than being determined from health impact.

Acknowledging these problems, one option for a better impact assessment process is the model of Risk Assessment. Using the classic steps of hazard identification, comparison of dose-response assessment and exposure assessment, leading to risk characterisation and risk management, the risk assessment paradigm attempts to overcome the lack of information regarding exposure and effects.

After a brief reference to risk assessment, the core of this presentation is spent in detailing a proposed method for an applicable means of Health Impact Assessment (HIA). The basic methodology shows increased attention to specific issues of location and population, since sensitive areas and groups may influence population and individual level health impact.

Six steps of the proposed approach can be summarised in terms of:

1. *Description of the study area* (physical conditions, existing pollution sources, use of area, natural resources and demography).
2. *Identification of relevant environmental changes.*
3. *Identification and quantification of exposure and internal dose.*
4. *Identification of expected health effects.*
5. *Assessment of health effects of planned situation.*
6. *Conclusions and mitigating factors* (options include limitation emissions or exposure, medical infrastructure).

In addition to these steps, *monitoring and post-project evaluation* is emphasised as an often neglected but important step in order to following-up the actual health effects of the project and improving health risk assessment methods. The entire process is noted as a complex, multistep procedure with multiple uncertainties, but with the potential to avoid the frequently erroneous and oversimplified health impact assessments that are being carried out as part of EIA today.

The contribution on **'Can Ecological Taxes Play a Role in Diminishing the Health Impacts of Waste Management?'** by Mr. Chris Steenwegen provides a comprehensive review of the role of economic instruments, and in particular ecotaxes, as a tool to improve waste management practices. As a dynamic tool suitable for non-point source pollution, ecotaxes could potentially discourage least desirable practices, fill the cost gap between recovery and recycling, encourage recovery and recycling and encourage prevention efforts.

In developing these themes, awareness of health impact of waste management is not referred to. Potential health benefits from ecotaxes are not directly addressed, but are implicit in the motivation to reduce waste, with ecotaxes referred to as a possible tool to influence consumer choice relating to harmful products such as batteries. The presentation focuses on experience in Belgium in relation to the implementation of ecotaxes, and their experience and potential influence on waste management practices including recycling, industrial packaging and batteries.

George Kamizoulis provides the last contribution to this section with a paper on the '**Co-ordinated Regional Action for the Reduction of Solid Waste Pollution in the Framework of the Mediterranean Action Plan**'. An overview is provided of WHO's role within the UN contribution to the larger structure of the Mediterranean Action Plan, having centres for research and planning in Tunisia, Barcelona, Marseille, Athens, France and Croatia which are involved with protection of the Mediterranean Sea against pollution.

Within this framework, awareness of health impact of waste management is only indirectly addressed through lists of issues that WHO is involved with which relate to health and pollution, including the urban environment (e.g. municipal sewerage, urban solid waste and air pollution), and industrial development (e.g. TPB's organochlorines, heavy metals). Assigned national targets and regional activities are listed, with associated time frames within which these objectives should be met. It is acknowledged that, according to the current situation, such objectives for decreasing environmental and health impact are unlikely to be met, but are useful as appropriate goals to work toward. Specific details of WHO's role in supporting these proposals are not given.

## 5. Case Studies

The first contribution in this section is by Gavin ten Tusscher *et al.* It is titled '**A Local Increased Incidence of Orofacial Clefts in Amsterdam: The Result of Open Combustion of Chemicals?**'. The paper is aimed at both providing an overview of general aspects of congenital abnormalities associated with waste, as well as introducing the relation between pollution and malformation. By introducing the basic stages of foetal development, the link is made between the timing of the environmental insult and the resulting congenital malformation.

Three major groups of defects are distinguished according to the stage of development:

i) neural tube defects - suggesting insult during the first 3 weeks of life;
ii) damage occurring between 3-9 weeks, corresponding to the period of organogenesis and sensitive to high-dose exposure. Associated malformations include the eye, heart, skeleton and palate defects;

iii) functional abnormalities occurring between 12-30 weeks associated with low-dose exposure, and leading to functional, behavioural and hormonal imbalance.

The paper focuses on congenital abnormalities relating to landfill sites and emphasises two key points. First, that the congenital malformations associated with landfill sites are *midline defects.* Midline defects include gastroschisis, spina bifida, sexual abnormalities, congenital heart disease, cleft palate and neural tube defects. In addition, there are findings to suggest congenital abnormalities related to exposure to landfills, are also associated with cancer later in adult life, which is plausible in relation to the potential effects of the chemicals involved.

The paper further provides a presentation of an epidemiological study of the increased incidence of cleft palate associated with a poorly regulated open incinerator occurring during the 1960s. The study involves a comparison of an exposed and less-exposed site in Amsterdam.

This presentation makes an overt focus on awareness of health impact of the waste management practice of incineration. Retrospective epidemiological techniques are used relating exposure and effects to determine the strength of the relationship between exposure to incinerator emissions and the health effects of orofacial clefts (cleft lip +/- cleft palate). The study is introduced by providing a historical background of the site, a comparison of the clinics and possible confounding factors, and to what extent they were corrected for.

The findings of the study demonstrate a sharp peak in incidence of orofacial defects after incineration began. These are associated with a definite locational pattern along a corridor of wind-flow from the incinerator. The biological plausibility of such a relationship is considered in terms of the knowledge that TCDD dioxin is known to cause cleft palate in mice, prompting the proposal that the mechanism of effect of a substance such as dioxin is through inhibition of palate fusion. In addition there is a historical increased incidence of cleft palate following exposure to Agent Orange in Vietnam.

The conclusion of the study begins by highlighting the difficulty of showing a cause-effect relationship, but notes that *'the unnatural trend of the incidence of non-syndromal orofacial defects at Zeeburg maternity clinic for the years 1960-1969 indicates that the open chemical combustions at Zeeburg resulted in a local increased incidence of orofacial defects.'*

The paper by Nik Van Larebeke, of Ghent University in Belgium is called **'Health Effects of a Household Waste Incinerator near Wilrijk, Belgium'**. This is based on a case study assessing the possibility of health impacts of an incinerator in Belgium. The research and findings presented raise several interesting points regarding awareness of health impacts of waste management.

First, the research undertaken in the region of the incinerator in Belgium was the work of a special commission that was set up due to *public concern* regarding a cluster of congenital anomalies in the Neerland district near to the Wilrijk incinerator. Local public concern had come to the attention of journalists, who in turn raised political interest in the issue, which resulted in a health study. Public awareness and concern regarding congenital abnormalities as health impacts of waste management is emphasised as a different and important contribution to increase political awareness of health impacts.

The findings of the study raise interesting issues regarding methods available for researching the link between health impact and waste management. Several different groups were studied in an effort to seek a relatively unexposed control group for comparison with the district of concern. Initial comparisons were made with a nearby region in Flanders, followed by comparison with the whole of Flanders, and also a district further to the west of Flanders. Despite this effort, it was recognised that it is very difficult to find a relatively clean control group for comparison in Flanders. This is related to the wide dispersion of pollution and the fact that exposure to contaminants of concern comes from food which is distributed throughout the region.

Findings of the studies relate to the following range of health outcomes:

- *Chromosomal aberrations:* no difference between twenty-four children in Neerland and twenty children from another area also near Antwerp.
- *Perinatal death:* no difference between Neerland and Flanders as a whole.

- *Congenital malformations*: slight increase in Neerland compared to Flanders as a whole (Odds Ratio =1.3) but this was not statistically significant. A non-significant increase in children born to mothers living in Neerland compared to children born in the same clinic to mothers who lived elsewhere.
- *Multiple pregnancies*: statistically significant increase in Neerland compared to the whole of Flanders, with an Odds Ratio of 2.6.
  There was no relation found between duration of residence of the parents in the Neerland area and the occurrence of congenital malformations or multiple pregnancies.
- *Failure at school:* no difference in the Neerland area compared to a nearby commune.
- *General health status:* increased prevalence of recurrent common colds was observed in the 3rd maternal class.

It was not possible to draw conclusions as to the health effects of the incinerator at Wilrijk, because data on many aspects of health are lacking, and comparisons are between regions that barely differ in their exposure.

Van Larebeke also puts emphasis on the concept of *chemical hygiene.* Drawing on his experience with cancers of environmental origin, the scale of human health impact due to chemical substances was highlighted by noting that 10 per cent of chemicals have some carcinogenic activity, and 2 per cent have endocrine function.

In response to the scale of this problem and the huge uncertainties faced in understanding it, it is very difficult to make priorities or choices in terms of what is acceptable as regards human health and well-being. With reference to the success of biological hygiene as a public health initiative during the past century, Nik Van Larebeke's conclusion was that, in order to arrive at true prevention, exposure to as many agents as possible must be lowered through concerted efforts to achieve *chemical hygiene* in our society.

The final case study is by Gesa Staats de Yanes and Vyvyan Howard. It addresses **'Impact of Inadequate or Negligent Waste Disposal on Wildlife and Domestic Animals: Relevance for Human Health'**. The paper makes explicit the links between the health impact of humans and the health effects on domestic animals of waste management and chemical pollution.

Attention is drawn to the contribution that environmental damage makes to disrupting human health in terms of total physical, social and psychological well-being. Links are made between waste-induced environmental degradation and the health impacts on wildlife and domestic animals, both of which are directly linked with human health. Not only can adverse health effects in wildlife due to environmental damage trigger necessary research in humans, but wildlife can also act as indicator species for contamination, domestic animal effects can directly contribute to human exposure through animal food products. Substances of concern relating to waste are listed and noted to reflect similar lists for humans. These include persistent organohalogens, heavy metals, pharmaceuticals, plasticisers, and organo-tin compounds.

Examples of various outbreaks and striking incidences of health effects in wildlife are provided. It is noted that the aquatic food web includes several species at high risk, reflecting lipophilic bio-accumulation of substances such as persistent organohalogens, with animals at the top of the food chain, such as polar bears and killer whales, at particular risk, as they eat high fat content fish and seals. This is relevant for humans, who are also at the top of the food chain.

PCBs are used as an example of widely dispersed persistent organohalogens which, despite increasingly strict regulations in countries such as Germany, are still in production in some countries today. The properties of PCBs determine their volatilisation from highly polluted areas, atmospheric transport and condensation into the final sink of open oceans. These substances are now accumulating in increasing concentrations in open oceans, posing a risk to both marine ecosystems and humans. Concern over this type of health impact has increased after epidemiological studies showed worrying levels of PCBs in populations with a high intake of marine animal fats such as the Inuit Indian and Fisherman studies in both Sweden and the Great Lakes.

The potential role of monitoring wildlife for time trends and regional trends in reproductive success, general health effects and body burden of hazardous substances is outlined. The high sensitivity of indicator species, such as fish, to detect obvious, easily detectable trends is also addressed, which could be used, for example, in detecting oestrogenic substances downstream from sewage plants or industrial sites. These indicators are noted as having a potentially greater sensitivity than the comparably lower sensitivity of other analytical and sampling methods.

Finally, domestic animals are highlighted as a major source of exposure to contamination in humans. Food of animal origin was noted as a major source of intake of organohalogens in man, with milk being one product that is well monitored, but other animal products under less control. Routes of contamination specific to animals include sewage sludge, incineration and fish. The potential repercussions of diluting and dispersing contaminated material that domestic animals are then exposed to was highlighted as a very dangerous practice, exemplified by a recent case of importing citrus pulp from Brazil which resulted in dangerous pesticide dispersal. Waste-related health effects in domestic animals are also noted as being of particular concern to humans when the exposure is through the ambient environment shared by humans.

## 6. Conclusions

The papers collected in these proceedings are the result of presentations given at a seminar on 'Health Impacts of Waste Management Policies' in Kos (Greece) during the period November 12-14, 1998. During the seminar discussions on a number of themes recurred, and are summarised here as crossover issues relating to the health-waste management interface.

### *The difference between potential technological capacity and actual performance.*

Technological means are important for solving environmental problems, but there is need to be realistic about their limitations. The difference between the theoretical capacity of lowering emissions from incinerators and what is actually emitted can result in important impacts on human health and this reality should be allowed for in any decision.

***The Burden of Proof argument and the precautionary principle.***

The discussion reflects an important debate in environmental health regarding whether the 'burden of proof' regarding health impact should be reassessed. Currently the evidence/proof needed to introduce a product or process is much less than the evidence/proof needed to remove it. This is because the 'burden of proof' lies with those who need to 'prove' that health impacts exist before being able to remove the cause of the problem. The contrasting scenario would involve the 'burden of proof' of safety resting with the producers.

The major arguments for reconsidering this situation focus on the need for precaution in the face of the inherent uncertainties and limitations of science when attempting to prove health impact. Contrasts are made with the level of certainty required by epidemiologists and toxicologists (e.g. when determining the need for intervention to protect health), with our willingness to accept high levels of uncertainties in other aspects of our daily lives relating to ambient environmental exposure. Enlarging on the earlier proposal for *chemical hygiene* and the reality that we are not just considering one substance but thousands, it is argued that *'chemicals should be considered dangerous until proven otherwise'*. As with the historical approach to achieving improved biological hygiene, it is proposed that we should invest in controlling the use of chemicals in a precautionary manner.

An opposing view argues against shifting the 'burden of proof' to the producer. This view highlights the risk of 'problem exchange' as an argument against lowering the burden of proof needed to remove a substance. Market forces and consumer demand mean that any banned product will be replaced and the new product may be equally as bad. Furthermore, a precautionary approach to new products may mean that important (potentially environmentally- and health-protective) innovations are not made available to the public. Risk is referred to again as relatively unavoidable in our society, and it is emphasised that attention should be focused on identification of and intervention in avoidable risks.

A further viewpoint is that additional ways should be sought to motivate producers to remove dangerous substances, beyond just waiting for high level of proof of their harm.

In the interim, producers should be taxed, or warned of imminent banning of dangerous substances in order to motivate them to develop more environmentally safe technology.

### *Hazard versus Risk Assessment - gaining contributions from tools available.*

References to *risk assessment* as a predictive means to determine health effects are contrasted against epidemiological studies which give a *hazard assessment* of the relationship between the exposure to a hazard and health impact in terms of clinical symptoms and pathology which have actually occurred in human populations. This approach is noted as providing more important additional information than other predictive methods, but was seen as confrontational for decision-makers and politicians, since it is politically emotive and demands action. Such action is difficult for politicians to take since the health benefits of intervention are likely to be difficult to measure and to occur outside the short time-scales that politicians work within.

A related comment is made that, whether from hazard or risk assessment, valuable information is now available regarding environmental health impacts from many sources. There should be better international harmonisation and exchange of this information to avoid redundancy and repetition, and speed decision-making.

### *The behavioural dimension of increasing awareness and changing attitudes.*

This theme, raised in response to the variety of theoretical solutions that are proposed, serves as a reminder that the proposed outcomes are going to be very difficult to achieve without being accompanied by a change in the behaviour and attitude of society. This is also related to the general theme of awareness of health impact and the problem that, without a change in attitude and behaviour, awareness itself may not lead to real action to protect health and the environment.

This theme recurs in Polyxeni Nicolopoulou-Stamati's comments regarding awareness and capacity for change within a group such as that present at the seminar. She points out the tendency for individuals to retain their own professional viewpoints without truly interacting with other ideas to broader their view, or develop abstract, innovative thinking about the problems under discussion and how to address them in practice.

***Time-lag and intergenerational health effects - further impetus for precaution.***

At its close, the discussion re-emphasised the need for precaution in the face of the problem of time-lag when considering environmental health issues. This is evident in the time taken for policy and legislation on intervention to be implemented. This problem is compounded since, in addition to intervention delays, there is a time-lag between the timing of an environmental insult, and the resulting health effects. These can occur in both children or adults over time, including through reproductive and genetic effects on the next generation.

This issue and its fundamental importance to the foetus, infants, and the children of coming generations led to a final re-emphasis, iterated by Dr. Howard, of the need for the *prioritisation of the child and infant in all regulatory procedures* regarding chemicals. Despite its obvious importance, this remains neglected in our existing assessment systems and regulatory institutions.

## References

Dolk, H., Vrijheid, M., Armstrong, B., Abramsky, L., Bianchi, F., Garne, E., Nelen, V., Robert, E., Scott, J.E., Stone, D., and Tenconi R. (1998) Risk of congenital anomalies near hazardous waste landfill sites in Europe: the EUROHAZCON study, *Lancet* **352 (9126)**, 423-7.

REHW (1998) Landfills are dangerous, *Rachel's Environment and Health Weekly* **#617**, September 24, http://www.rachel.org/.

# THE WASTE MANAGEMENT AND THE HEALTH SCENE

# PERSISTENT ORGANIC CHEMICAL POLLUTION: AN INTRODUCTION

C.V. HOWARD[1]
G. STAATS DE YANES[2]
P. NICOLOPOULOU-STAMATI[3]
[1]*University of Liverpool*
*Fetal & Infant Toxico-Pathology*
*P.O. Box 147*
*L69 7ZA Liverpool*
*UNITED KINGDOM*
[2]*WHO-Centre*
*Tierärztlichen Hochschule Hannover*
*Bünteweg 2*
*D-30559 Hannover*
*GERMANY*
[3]*National and Capodistrian University of Athens*
*Medical School, Department of Pathology*
*75, Micres Ajias, GOYDI*
*11527 Athens*
*GREECE*

## Summary

The organic chemical industry, in the space of half a century, has produced millions of tons of persistent carbon-based compounds which can now be found in every part of the globe and in the body fat of every living creature. These compounds can be either



*P. Nicolopoulou-Stamati et al. (eds.), Health Impacts of Waste Management Policies*, 29–40.

intentionally released products (such as DDT), or unintentionally released as industrial chemical by-products (such as the dioxin-like substances). The majority of the dioxins and furans that have been introduced into the environment have come about as a result of the incineration of municipal and clinical waste, which contains high levels of halogenated compounds and heavy metals. Persistent organic pollutants (POPs) are lipophilic and difficult to metabolise, and therefore they bioconcentrate in the body over time and biomagnify up the food web.

Recent research has shown for some POPs, such as polychlorinated biphenyls (PCBs) and dioxin-like substances, that human body burdens in a proportion of the populations of developed countries are already too high for the safety of the next generations. Adverse effects on the intelligence, immune status and hormonal balance of infants born to mothers with the highest body burdens have been measured.

Thus there is an urgent requirement for the elimination of the most problematic persistent substances, or their precursors, from the waste stream and hence the biosphere. There are some interesting developments in the field of biodegradable polymers, research into which need to be both supported and extended.

The aim of this chapter is to provide the reader with an overview of the origins of and contributors to global persistent organic pollution so that they can then set the rest of the information in this book in context. In addition the reader should be better able to critically weigh the evidence produced by contributors to this book from various sides of the argument.

## 1. Introduction

The past five decades has seen the emergence of whole new groups of man-made bulk organic chemicals which have been found to persist in the biosphere. Their persistence poses real problems for those involved in waste disposal. We all carry traces of these chemicals in our bodies and it is now conservatively estimated that the average person in the economically-developed countries has between three hundred and five hundred discernable residues (Howard, 1997). These chemicals would not have been detected fifty years ago because they were not being manufactured in any appreciable amounts and do not occur naturally. The effect of such a mixture is completely unknown and, indeed, unmeasureable by current technology.

## 2. Organohalogens - an Example of a Group of Persistent Organic Pollutants Causing Problems to Waste Management

Organohalogens are substances containing chemically combined halogen atoms and carbon. The halogens consist of fluorine, chlorine, bromine and iodine. They first emerged as convenient by-products of the expanding chlorine industry in the 1930's. The chemical properties of organochlorines (a specific family of organohalides), including low flammability, chemical stability and apparent lack of immediate toxicity to humans, made them very desirable for industrial use. As a result there are now some eleven thousand organochlorines which are known to be produced and used commercially for products as diverse as pesticides, plastics, solvents, lubricants and refrigerants (Johnston and McCrea, 1992). Organobromine compounds are known to have many similar properties.

Organochlorines do occur naturally in the environment, but only at very low levels. About two thousand compounds are known to be produced by living organisms which contain chlorine, or its related elements iodine, bromine or fluorine (Gribble, 1994). Chloromethane, which is produced by marine algae, is the only natural organochlorine to occur in any significant quantity (Naumann, 1993), and may play a part in regulating the ozone layer. The naturally-occurring organochlorines do not include highly chlorinated hydrocarbons. The latter are generally highly lipophilic and persistent substances which accumulate in the environment and are only produced as synthetic man-made chemicals (Henschler, 1994).

The same properties that made organochlorines desirable to chemical industry have created widespread environmental problems. Once introduced into the environment, the stability of many organohalides means they degrade very slowly. This is because the carbon-halide bond in these chemicals is generally very strong and resists being broken down by normal biochemical and physical processes. Consequently, some organochlorines may take 100 years or more to break down completely into harmless inorganic salts, whilst others do not degrade to any appreciable extent at all. Moreover, when organohalides do break down, they usually produce other organohalides - the carbon-halogen chemical bond remaining intact as part of another compound - and these are often more toxic and far more hazardous than the original substance. The number of unidentified organohalides produced in this way is believed to be vast.

Some organohalides, such as the refrigerants chloro-fluoro-carbons (CFCs), and solvents, such as chloroform, are volatile and tend to evaporate into the atmosphere, where they slowly break down. In the upper atmosphere some organohalogens act as powerful ozone depleters, while others may degrade in the lower atmosphere. All of them can be transported long distances by air currents and may eventually be deposited in the surface waters of rivers, lakes or seas. Other less volatile organochlorines, including polychlorinated biphenyls (PCBs), dioxins and many pesticides, can be transported in air and water currents or become bound up in soil or sediments. Since organohalides can be transported in air and water currents, many have become globally ubiquitous, from the deep sea-bed to the stratosphere, from the Arctic to the Antarctic. The production of organohalides from industry far outstrips the rate at which they are broken down in the environment into harmless chemicals. This means there is an ever-increasing load of organohalides being added to the environment each year.

Another major feature of organohalides is their tendency to be strongly soluble in fat. They therefore are susceptible to undergoing 'bio-accumulation' over a lifetime and 'biomagnification' from the bottom to the top of the food web. Studies comparing the concentrations of dioxins in the water of the Great Lakes with those found in the top predator, the herring gull, found concentrations had increased by over 20,000,000 times. The half-life of dioxins in the body is estimated to be about ten years.

## 3. Human and Environmental Health Effects Associated with Organohalogens

The message from the latest research is that a proportion of members of the population already have enough of certain organochlorine pollutants in their bodies that, if they are (a) female, and (b) become pregnant. Mothers can pass on sufficient toxics to their babies across the placenta and in the breast milk to cause measurable adverse effects. The predominant effect has been found to be due to the exposure in the womb rather than through the breast milk. These effects include loss of intelligence, suppression of the immune system and interference with hormone systems in the body and are measured in a dose-related way to the mother's body burden (Lanting, 1999; Patandin, 1999). The rate at which dioxin-like substances transfer to the infant, as a function of duration of breastfeeding is shown in Figure 1. It is estimated that up to 1 per cent of the exposure up to the age of 25 can be transferred to the infant during breastfeeding for 6 months. Loss of cognition in offspring associated with maternal PCB body burden is shown in Figure 2.

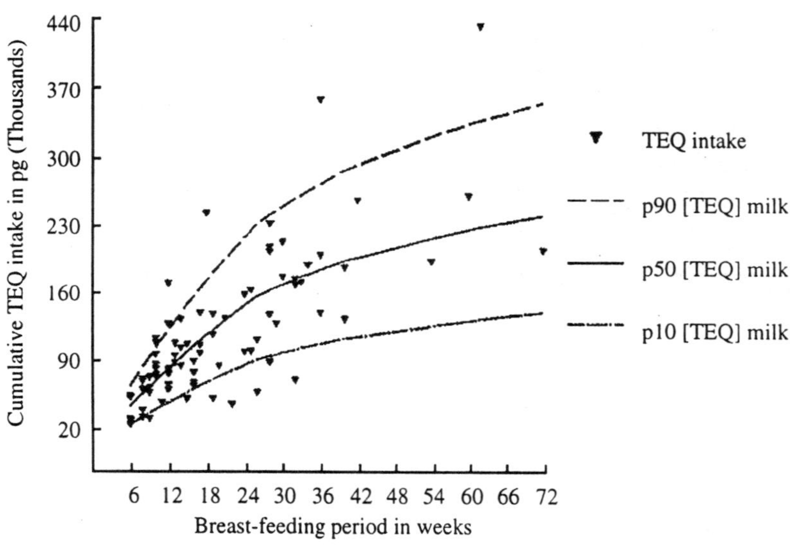


*Figure 1.* Cumulative intake of PCB and dioxin toxic equivalents (TEQs) as a function of breast feeding period (after Patandin, 1999).

Historically, when a widespread pollutant has been shown to pose a threat to human health, the regulatory authorities have tried to impose control by defining a tolerable daily intake (TDI), at which level it is judged that the risk of harm is acceptable. However, while this approach has some merit as a public health control measure when the pollutant doesn't build up in the body, it does not follow that TDIs can be logically applied to pollutants that persist and bio-accumulate.

Until recently, the recommended World Health Organisation TDI for dioxin-like substances was 10 pg I-TEQ/kg body wt/day. A recent Dutch Health Council report has recommended a ten-fold reduction in the TDI to 1 pg I-TEQ/kg body wt/day, based on the findings of Dutch scientists that state that adverse effects on the hormone status, immune status and neuro-behavioural development in infants can be significantly correlated with the mother's body burden of dioxin-like substances. The WHO has recently revised its TDI downwards. Currently best estimates of average daily intakes for dioxin-like substances are 2 pg I-TEQ/kg body wt/day in Holland and 3 pg I-TEQ/kg body wt/day in the UK. Intakes in breastfed babies are considerably higher than in adults, as shown for Germany in Table 1.

*Table 1.* I-TEQ values in morther's milk, North Rhine-Westfalia 1994, and daily intake by infants (Fürst *et al.*, 1995).

| **Mother's milk, n=50** | | | **Daily intake of I-TEQ** | | | | | |
|---|---|---|---|---|---|---|---|---|
| **pg/g lipid based** | | | **Total pg** | | | **pg/kg bw/day** | | |
| Med | Min | Max | Med | Min | Max | Med | Min | Max |
| 16.1 | 4.9 | 30.3 | 386 | 118 | 727 | 77 | 24 | 145 |

Basis: body weight (BW) 5 kg, milk amount 800 ml, lipid content 3 per cent.

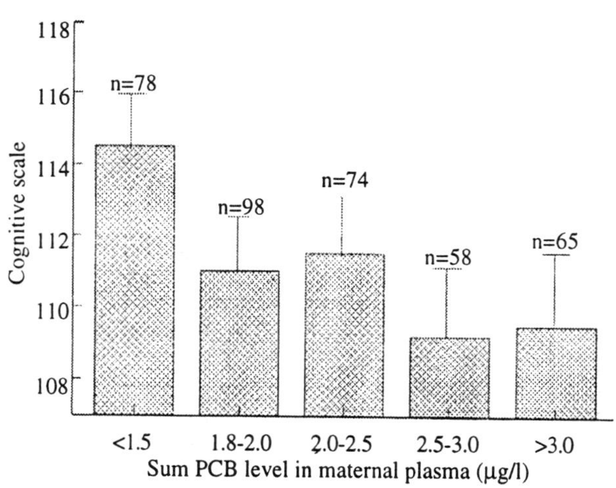


*Figure 2.* The association between the Dutch version of the Kaufman Assessment Battery for children and maternal PCB level (after Lanting, 1999).

Dr. Linda Birnbaum (1998), who is a senior official in the US EPA stated at 'Dioxin '98', in Stockholm, that 'Total Body Burden' is the most relevant metric to apply to human health, when dealing with persistent bio-accumulative chemicals. TCDD is avidly absorbed from the gastro-intestinal and respiratory tracts. Birnbaum confirmed that its most sensitive effects observed in multiple species appear to be developmental, including effects on the developing immune, nervous and reproductive systems. However, alterations have been noted in the adult immune systems and also in some biochemical indices. Among the most important observations in recent years is that of functional developmental toxicity; for examples, lifelong changes in behaviour as a result of exposure in the womb to low doses of dioxin-like substances.

Most importantly, Birnbaum pointed out that the endpoints of chronic and acute exposure are the same. In other words, it doesn't matter how a certain dose of dioxin gets into the body, the effects are identical. **Therefore, the total body burden (i.e. the total amount of dioxin in the body) is the single most relevant measurement that can be made**. Most current regulations, however, are based on the TDI, which Birnbaum acknowledged was less than adequate.

The most sensitive effects observed so far result from body burdens which are in the range of current human levels, which in the USA are on average 10 ng I-TEQ/kg body wt. One per cent of the population have total body burdens in the range 30-40 ng I-TEQ/kg body wt. Oxidative stress, which is associated with teratogenesis (foetal malformations), induction of enzymes and carcinogenesis, can occur at body burdens as low as 0.45 ng/kg body wt. In experiments, rats with a dioxin body burden of 100 ng I-TEQ/kg body wt were noted as having, at 18 months of age, a continuing reduction in allergic response, indicating that the immune system had been permanently altered.

Van Leeuwen and Younes (1998) (WHO Netherlands) have addressed the recent decision by the WHO to revise downwards the TDI for dioxin-like substances from 10 to between 1 to 4 pg WHO-TEQ/kg body wt/day. They stated that the International Association for Research in Cancer (IARC) had in February 1997 reclassified TCDD to a full Class 1 (definite) human carcinogen.

However, they acknowledged that subtle health effects in humans are currently occurring at an intake of between 1 to 3 pg I-TEQ/kg body wt/day (including PCB 2-3-times more). Therefore, the new WHO level cannot be regarded as a no-effect level. It is hoped that the daily intake will fall below 1 pg I-TEQ/kg body wt/day in most countries by the year 2003.

Van Leeuwen and Younes (1998) gave the following comparative table (Table 2) of measured effects versus body burdens in rats and the calculated body burdens (safety factor 2) in humans at the Dioxin '98 Conference in Stockholm.

*Table 2.* Measured effects versus body burdens of dioxin in different species (after Van Leeuwen and Younes, 1998).

| **Effect** | **Body burden ng/kg (ppt)** | |
|---|---|---|
| | **Rats** | **Human** |
| Reduced sperm count | 28 | 14 |
| Immunosuppression | 50 | 25 |
| Increased gonadal malformations | 73 | 37 |
| | **Monkeys** | **Human** |
| Neuro-behavioural deficits | 42 | 21 |
| Endometriosis | 42 | 21 |

This, compared with Birnbaum's data of an average USA body burden 10 ng I-TEQ/kg body wt with 1 per cent having as high as 30-40 ng I-TEQ/kg body weight, makes alarming reading and it is clear that, at current levels of exposure, a proportion of the human race is already exposed to the extent that adverse effects are occurring.

## 4. Waste Disposal Problems Associated with Organohalogens

Many of the ephemeral artefacts of our 'throw away' society are made from organohalogen compounds. It is estimated that 30 per cent of the current annual global chlorine production of 40,000,000 tonnes goes into the production of polyvinyl chloride (PVC). It is to be found literally everywhere in plastic toys, packaging, paints, wallcoverings, flooring, electrical goods - the list is endless. When such products reach the end of their life, which may be only a few days in the case of a shopping bag, plastic bottle or disposable razor, they become part of the waste stream. The proportion of plastic in household and industrial waste has increased inexorably over the past decades. This poses a problem for waste disposal authorities, because it is generally not biodegradable, but can occupy considerable volume.

An additional hazard is that if organohalide products become involved in combustion processes, as for example each time a building or landfill site catches fire, a new set of highly toxic compounds is formed. Of these, the dioxins have been the most widely studied and their toxicity to humans is discussed in the next section. The widespread use of the mass incineration of municipal household waste and clinical waste in the USA and many European countries has been attributed to have caused between 50 per cent and 80 per cent of the total dioxin contamination of land. This has now led to the closure of most municipal and clinical waste incinerators in Europe and the development of a new generation of high capacity incinerators with improved temperature control and gas cleaning technology. However, although this new generation of incinerators is, thankfully, an improvement over the previous models, there are still many questions about where the ashes they produce are to be deposited and how toxic they remain. In addition, on a more local basis, the production of respirable particulate pollution and its health impacts remain to be investigated. In the vicinity of point sources, concentrations may reach levels up to a factor of ten higher than found at sites remote from industrial activity. In Table 3 this is compared to other intakes.

*Table 3.* Comparative daily intake data on dioxins TEQ associated with a variety of sources (Liem, 1999).

| | pg/kg/day |
|---|---|
| Average | 2-3 |
| MWI | 5-10 |
| Baby | 200 |
| Seveso | 10-100 |
| Yusho | 158,000 |

In the last few decades, several accidents causing excess exposure of humans to dioxin related compounds have been reported. Well-known examples are exposure of the local population at Seveso, and from fires in PCB-filled electrical equipment. High exposure may also be caused by food items accidentally contaminated. Known examples are the contamination of edible oil, such as the Yusho (Japan) and Yu-Cheng (Taiwan) food poisoning. Occupational activities in which 2,3,7,8-TCDD and related compounds are unintentionally produced, such as waste incineration or production of certain pesticides or chemicals, may also result in an additional human exposure.

Clearly, incineration and landfilling are 'end of pipe' solutions to the waste problem, each with their own associated problems. Furthermore, they give the message to the producers of problematic toxic waste products that it is 'business as usual' and there is no need to seek out new technologies to replace the old ones with less environmentally-damaging alternatives.

## 5. Conclusions

An example has been given of a group of organohalide chemicals, the organochlorines, which have been mass produced on a global scale for some fifty years and in that time have become widespread on a planetary scale. Despite knowledge that these have effects on both human and environmental health, the world production of chlorine continues to rise.

Measurements of human health, particularly for those at the beginning of life, indicate that at current body burdens adverse effects can be measured. There is a clear indication that the global production of dioxin-like substances must be reduced urgently. Most organochlorine products can be converted into toxic products of incomplete combustion, including dioxins, if intentionally or accidentally involved in a combustion process. Therefore there is already a massive global store of organochlorine products, which will eventually become waste, with the potential to contribute to the current planetary burden of toxic persistent organochlorine pollutants.

The consequences for waste management policy are severe. A sensible approach will be to identify those groups of chemical compounds that do cause major problems to society in general, and the waste disposal industry in particular, and timetable the sunsetting of their production to realistic but tight deadlines. This will fire the research needed to find viable replacements, which in their turn must be assessed for persistence, bio-accumulation and toxicity before being licensed. Until such phaseouts are achieved, it is very important to attempt to separate the toxins from the waste stream and keep them under control, possibly by binding them into stable matrices. However this must be seen as a stop-gap measure while awaiting the phasing out of the production of those organics which are persistent and bio-accumulative.

Thankfully, there are technological advances which offer some hope. For example, there is a new method of extruding polyvinyl alcohol (PVA). Although many decades of research have been spent developing PVA it was hitherto unsatisfactory for melt-processing, because it degrades below its melting point. These problems have now been overcome and because PVA is a truly biodegradable polymer for which environmentally neutral disposal options exist, this represents a genuine advance. In addition, the only plasticisers that need to be added to PVA are water and food-grade glycerine, neither of which have any known problems of hormone mimicry associated with some phthalate esters used in the softening of PVC. Other potentially interesting biodegradable polymers are currently being researched, for example the polycaprolactans and polylactic acids. Governments need to examine the restructuring of the tax system to encourage such technological research and to discourage the use of products that continue to cause problems long after they have outlived their useful life.

## Acknowledgement

The authors would like to thank Ms. V. Mountford for her detailed proof reading of the manuscript.

## References

Birnbaum, L.S. (1998) Sensitive non-carcinogenic effects of TCDD in animals, *Organohalogen Compounds* **38**, 291-294, ISBN 91-89192-07-9.

Fürst, P. (1995) *Jahresbericht des Chemischen Landes- und Staatlichen Veterinär Untersuchungsamtes*, Münster, Nordrhein Westfalen, Germany. (in German)

Gribble, G.W. (1994) The natural production of chlorinated compounds, *Environ. Sci. Technol.* **28** **(7)**, 310A-318A.

Henschler, D. (1994) Toxicity of organic compounds: Effects of the introduction of chlorine in organic molecules, *Angew. Chem. Int. Ed. Engl.* **33**, 1920-1935.

Howard, C.V. (1997) Synergistic effects of chemical mixtures. Can we rely on traditional toxicology? *The Ecologist* **27**, 192-195.

Johnston, P.J., and McCrea, I. (1992) *Death in Small Doses*, Greenpeace International, ISBN 1871532 61 2.

Lanting, C.I. (1999) *Effects of Perinatal PCB and Dioxin Exposure and Early Feeding Mode on Child Development*, PhD Thesis, Printpartners Ipskamp B.V., Enschede, ISBN 90-367-1002-2.

Liem, A.K.D. (1999) Dioxins and dioxin-like PCBs in foodstuffs. Levels and trends, *Organohalogen Compounds* **44**, 1-4.

Naumann, K. (1993) Chlorchemie der Natur, *Chemie in unserer Zeit* **27** (**1**), 33-41. (in German)

Patandin, S. (1999) *Effects of Environmental Exposure to Polychlorinated Biphenyls and Dioxins on Growth and Development in Young Children*, PhD Thesis, Microweb, Saasveld, ISBN 90-9012306-7.

Van Leeuwen, F.X.R, and Younes, M. (1998) WHO revises the Tolerable Daily Intake (TDI) for dioxins, *Organohalogen Compounds* **38**, 295-296, ISBN 91-89192-07-9.

# THE CHALLENGE TO ACHIEVE BETTER LANDFILLS WHERE ONLY DUMPS ARE ACHIEVED NOW: AN ANTHOLOGY

P. RUSHBROOK
*Regional Advisor, Waste Management*
*WHO Rome Operational Division*
*Via Francesco Crispi 10*
*00187 Rome*
*ITALY*

**Summary**

All around the world the inadequate, unsafe and unhealthy open dumping of solid waste remains the most widely used waste disposal method. It thrives on the mistaken belief that it is the cheapest disposal method and the only one possible in places with difficult economic and social conditions. It is argued that this belief need not be true.

In general, clean and healthy living conditions in cities, towns and villages cannot be achieved without reliable and regular waste collection and disposal. In past years much effort has been expended in the more progressive cities and towns to improve urban collection services. They should now be encouraged direct in their attention towards improving the standard of landfill disposal. Open dumping is prevalent in around one hundred and seventy-five countries out of about two hundred sovereign states and distinct territories in total. It has become more and more obvious that it is no longer realistic simply to remove the potential health risks posed by waste from city streets only to accumulate them at an open dump in a nearby suburb or rural area. No amount of careful



*P. Nicolopoulou-Stamati et al. (eds.), Health Impacts of Waste Management Policies,* 41–56.

collection or waste treatment will reduce the hazards to health and the environment posed by disposal, if the final resting place for waste is an open dump. Open dumping is a generator of ill-health.

## 1. Health Effects

In general, four categories of health effects may occur at poorly designed or operated waste disposal sites:

1. Direct physical harm arising from the collapse of unstable slopes of waste, explosions and fires, asphyxiation, waste-related transport accidents, falls and musculo-skeletal injuries.
2. Bacteriological and protozoal pathogens and similar infective agents arising from the biological contamination of waste and their subsequent infective transmission to a host. Transmission routes via hand to mouth and hand to food to mouth are most common among waste workers and scavengers, while contamination of water supply or uptake through the food chain could affect the general public.
3. Similar transmission routes may apply to chemical contaminants from waste affecting target organs or regulatory and control functions within the body. The chemical inducement of cancers is also a theoretical possibility.
4. The consequences of chemical or microbiological contaminants on reproduction, notably still-birth, low birthweights or specific birth defects, are also known. There have also been incidents of ill-health and death from exposure to dumped organic chemical compounds and even radioactive materials.

In the majority of middle- and lower-income countries the primary objective of the municipal waste service is still seen as that of protecting public health. As such, what limited resources that are available to the waste services in municipalities are directed towards maintaining waste collection, especially from residential areas. It is the presence of uncollected waste lying for a long period of time close to residential areas that presents the greatest threat to public health. It is a constant concern of waste managers in many cities where money, vehicles and spare parts are in short supply, and delays and breakdowns can significantly reduce the area of the town that receives a waste collection service.

With the understandable public health pre-occupation with collection, improvements to waste disposal are, correspondingly, a lower priority. Only those improvements that require little or no new money or resources stand a chance of being considered in most of the one hundred and seventy-five or so lower- and middle-income countries. Open dumping remains the most widespread disposal method and, except in only a minority of places, receives little or no management attention by the municipality. 'Out of sight, out of mind' is often the attitude encountered.

The motivation to increase the prevailing standards of waste management in lower- and middle-income countries to protect the environment is a relatively new concept in many places. Whilst waste managers and the general public are becoming more knowledgeable about environmental damage (and its potential secondary effects on human health), the realities dictated by the amount of materials and funds locally available means that attempts to raise waste standards have to be tempered by what is locally sustainable. This means that meaningful efforts to upgrade operational standards in a waste service should be a series of gradual, step-wise improvements whose incremental benefits become apparent over time. Great technological leaps are more than likely to fail.

## 2. From Open Dumping to Better Landfilling

Open dumping thrives because of the mistaken belief that it is the cheapest disposal method. It is inevitable that, if uncontrolled, the chemical and biological contaminants in waste will find their way back to man to affect health and productivity. Soluble or suspended contaminants in the liquid (leachate) from the waste will enter surface watercourses and the groundwater. Contamination may then directly affect drinking water supplies and/or the aquatic food chain. Grazing animals on dumps can pass on diseases via the terrestrial food chain, as well as via pests through infestation. Those living on or near a dump are also at risk from direct hand-to-mouth transfer of contamination and from inhalation of volatile compounds, bacterial spores and aerosols.

Recent programmes of assistance to municipalities have recognised the technical and financial difficulties in past attempts to leap directly from open dumping to sophisticated sanitary landfill. Such attempts have nearly always been found to be unsustainable by the local economy and local resources available. There are an increasing number of sophisticated sanitary landfills being constructed with donor grants or loans in, for example, Asia and the Balkans, which are subsequently run as open dumps because the waste managers' skills and the municipal organisations are not sufficiently developed to operate them any better. However, the absence of a sophisticated sanitary landfill in a municipality should not be a reason to avoid trying other, better land disposal techniques.

Some form of 'better landfill' can always be achieved, even in low-income countries, if local political will and waste manager commitment exists. Often significant improvements can be made by using the existing staff, equipment and finance available in a different way. Whenever it is possible to achieve, the resulting improved landfill should represent an improvement on open dumping. Such an achievement should be commended whenever it occurs, not derided as a lowly intermediate solution.

The distinguishing advantages that all better landfill operations have, to a lesser or greater extent, over open dumps are:

- partial or full geological isolation of waste from the environment;
- civil engineering preparations, preferably before the site receives waste;
- the ability of the staff at the site to control the waste disposal operation;
- an organised deposit of waste in a small working area which, preferably, is spread, compacted and covered daily.

It should be emphasised that no one should expect the immediate adoption and implementation of a sophisticated and highly mechanised landfill operation. What is important is to recognise those parts of the present land disposal operation that are unsanitary and to look for ways to improve them with local sources. Recent work within the WHO, taking into account the earlier views of others, has led to the suggestion of a 'pathway' to upgrade, over time, the quality of municipal waste landfill sites:

### *Stage 1: Open Dumping to 'Controlled Dumping'*

This involves three changes. First, the reduction in the working area of the site to a more manageable size (say, 2 ha for a modest sized city of 500,000 inhabitants) and the covering with soil, sand or any other convenient material, of all unneeded areas of the site. Second, stopping fires, and third, agreeing 'rules' for on-site co-operation with scavengers if they cannot be removed completely.

None of these controlled dumping measures represent a major increase in the amount of resources used at an open dump. The advantage is that they introduce the philosophy of 'control' and 'isolation' into the waste disposal operation. Since this first incremental step is relatively small, the risk of failure perceived by a landfill manager can, equally, be argued to be small. In this situation, outside technical assistance can provide strong support for waste managers in the first few weeks after introducing changes. This approach was recently proposed as part of a continuing programme of work in Turkmenistan. A technical advisor worked in collaboration with a municipal landfill operator, local civil engineering designers and university engineering lecturers to encourage the implementation of a set of simple operating improvements to the existing open dump.

### *Stage 2: Controlled Dumping to 'Engineered Landfill'*

This second stage along the pathway involves the gradual adoption of engineering techniques to: restrict and avoid surface water entering the waste; extract and spread soil to cover wastes; gather leachate into lagoons; spread and compact waste into smaller layers; prepare new parts of the landfill with excavation equipment; and improve the isolation of waste from the surrounding geology. A clear sign that a municipality is progressing through this stage successfully is the routine development of detailed designs prior to new landfills being constructed, and the creation of tipping plans showing how a site will be filled with waste over its lifetime and how it will be finished off.

This stage represents the longest period in the evolution towards sophisticated landfill techniques. It encompasses the gradual accumulation of engineering expertise by those managers most closely associated with landfill operations. It may well take one generation of engineers to accumulate sufficient experience and confidence to progress through this stage of landfill development entirely. It is to those towns which are clearly within this stage of landfill development that specialised procurement, international study tours and technical engineering training are most suited. Extensive texts have also been published recently on appropriate landfill design and operation which are specifically targeted at assisting waste managers in this stage of landfill development (Diaz *et al.*, 1996; Rushbrook and Pugh, 1999).

A highly original approach has recently been adopted in South Africa which defines different levels of engineering preparation and operation at landfills depending on the site and location of individual sites (Government of South Africa, 1994).

### *Stage 3: Engineered Landfill to (Sophisticated) 'Sanitary Landfill'*

It has to be recognised that some communities and countries will not achieve this stage of landfill development in the foreseeable future. The progress towards a truly sanitary landfill, as recognised in the higher-income countries, involves the continuing refinement and increasing complexity of the engineering design and construction techniques begun in the engineered landfill stage. In addition, sanitary landfills are more likely to have the pre-planned installation of landfill gas control or utilisation measures, extensive environmental monitoring points and bore holes, a highly organised and trained work force, detailed record-keeping by the site office, and in some circumstances, on-site leachate treatment to supplement a leachate collection system.

It is important to appreciate that the sustained adoption of sophisticated sanitary landfills can only occur where the local economy can afford the higher levels of operational expenditure necessary, where waste managers are given professional status and authority commensurate with other engineering management roles, and where the advanced equipment and resources required to achieve high standards of operation are made available.

An overriding characteristic in communities operating sophisticated sanitary landfills is the ever-increasing social requirement of higher and higher environmental standards. Standards that become increasingly divorced from mere protection from credible health and environmental risks, to ones that reflect society's increasing intolerance with the concept of the landfill. There are very few examples of successful aid assistance provided by international agencies in this stage of landfill development. Typically, when a country or municipality can afford to adopt sanitary landfills, they are most likely to be able to buy in the necessary talent and resources directly from specialist public or private (sector) organisations.

## 3. Landfill 'Basic Truths'

Whether a city permits open dumping or operates highly engineered and sophisticated landfills, there are some common features (perhaps better to say 'basic truths') underlying all disposal to land options:

1. **Landfills are always going to be needed in any waste management strategy.** If someone claims otherwise then they must be congratulated for discovering perpetual motion.
2. **All waste in the ground will be acted upon by processes that will further its chemical, physical and microbiological decomposition.** If decomposition is not permitted to flourish then it is a storage site not a landfill.
3. **Since waste degrades, landfills should provide a suitable internal environment to make the products of decomposition less mobile, even if pre-treatment processes occur beforehand.** Where strategies are pursued that work against this restriction of the mobility of the products of degradation, then the disposal site will become a dump, not a landfill.
4. **All landfills, just like waste treatment processes, will have both a negative and positive impact on the environment.** Then again, all human intervention and development has both negative and positive effects. To deny this is a self-delusion.
5. **The intention should be for all land disposal sites to be, or become, well designed and engineered operations.** This is not an abstract concept, but one that requires political will and management commitment to realise. The kind of progress achieved relies on the physical and financial resources available to operate

the site, and the operational standards regarded as acceptable in each locality. (Rushbrook, 1998)

## 4. Prerequisites for Improvements in Landfill Operations

The prevailing opinion in many municipalities using open dumping is that local conditions are not conducive to developing a better operation. These may be political, social, technical or financial conditions, or a combination of two or more. Consequently, before a lasting improvement can be contemplated, this mindset has to be recognised, addressed and overcome, at least in part. This is what is meant by the prerequisites to achieving better landfill.

Seven prerequisites have been identified:

1. Political will and management commitment
2. Trust amongst all parties
3. Long-term sustainability
4. Gradual approach to landfill improvement
5. Relevant guidance
6. Countering risk aversion
7. Co-operative roles for enforcement and training.

Satisfying these prerequisites is neither an exact science nor an infallible art.

### *4.1. Political Will and Management Commitment*

No municipal service provided by a municipality or its public service enterprises exists in isolation from the control and decisions of the local elected representatives. No matter what political system prevails in a country or area, there is always one or more people empowered to make policy decisions regarding the municipal infrastructure, to allocate public funds and resources, and to justify the quality of life enjoyed by local citizens. The power to take policy decisions on a wide range of topics is a strong motivator in local and national politics. The power to take decisions on waste management is just one small part of this. Consequently, waste management is easily overlooked in the midst of all of the other demands competing for public resources, particularly in times of economic hardship and tight public-sector spending policies.

Little change to waste services can be achieved without a strong will on the part of the local politicians to see an improvement. It is therefore a crucial prerequisite to gain political support in advance of attempting to upgrade a waste collection or disposal service. This political will should manifest itself as the sustained allocation of additional finance and materials, possible legislative changes to help waste managers, and the firm support of the media and citizens for the improvements proposed by waste managers.

A highly successful example of sustained political will to improve an urban environment can be found in Curitiba, Brazil, where strong and inspired political involvement in environmental projects has been repeatedly affirmed, and public resources allocated, or obtained from other parties, to back the initiatives.

### *4.2. Trust Amongst All Parties*

One of the most difficult human virtues to restore once it has been lost is 'trust'. Once a waste collection service fails to collect waste regularly, or a waste disposal site is run as an open dump that is environmentally damaging and unsightly, then the trust of citizens in the municipal department is lost. If no public collection service or disposal site is available to commercial outlets they will set up their own dump sites or pay a contractor to take the waste away without too many questions being asked. The loss of trust for a municipal service creates, over time, a culture of self-sufficiency. Citizens burn or bury waste near their properties, or pay the private or informal sectors to take away waste when the accumulation of waste becomes too large and foul-smelling. Spontaneous informal dump sites become prevalent. A breakdown in trust is indicative of a waste system going out of control.

Even within a municipal organisation a lack of trust between departments is sometimes inevitable. The site workers on a landfill do not operate it as well as they could because they have wage complaints, or problems with the supply of fuel or spare parts. Municipalities often direct a greater proportion of resources to collection than disposal operations. Consequently, regular fluctuations in resources available to operate or upgrade and sustain landfills further erode the trust of landfill workers in the management of the waste service. There is often strong resistance within a municipality to agreeing to rely on a shared service which is to be provided by another municipality or agency. They are well aware of the problems they (and the other municipalities) encounter in making use of such a service and need considerable reassurance that relinquishing their self-sufficiency will not lead to greater difficulties in the future.

### *4.3. Long-Term Sustainability*

No-one has yet come up with a practical definition of sustainability in waste management; a definition that takes this notion out of the realms of a desirable political concept and into real life. Perhaps a working definition for sustainability in waste management could be:

> *'The achievement of a reasonably reliable waste service (collection, land disposal, etc.) that is of a reasonably acceptable standard to the local community, and reasonably affordable using chiefly local finance and resources, is probably a reasonably sustainable waste management system.'*

There is no practical benefit in developing a sophisticated landfill operation that cannot be sustained by a local municipality with the physical and financial resources it can provide in the long run.

A simplified example of the direct effect of the availability of local financial resources on the standard of a waste activity that can be sustained is presented in Table 4. Based on data drawn from actual situations, the table illustrates the levels of revenue available to run waste operations in a higher- and middle-income country.

It is evident that the sophistication of waste management that can be sustained financially is significantly greater in the higher-income nation (Country A) than the middle-income state (Country B). Even if one takes into account lower salaries, the obvious conclusion is that strict adherence to establishing, over the short and medium term, sophisticated landfills (or other expensive engineered technologies) in middle- or lower-income countries is probably not financially sustainable.

*Table 4.* A simplified example of the direct effect of the availability of local financial resources on waste management.

| **Country A – Higher-income Municipality** | | **Country B – Middle-income Municipality** | |
|---|---|---|---|
| Gross National Product (GNP) per person per year | US$ 20,000 | Gross National Product (GNP) per person per year | US$ 5,000 |
| Proportion of GNP per person spent on waste management | 0.5% | Proportion of GNP per person spent on waste management | 0.5% |
| Level of revenue available for waste per person per year | US$ 100 | Level of revenue available for waste per person per year | US$ 25 |
| For a municipal population of 100,000 this represents | US$ 10,000,000 | For a municipal population of 100,000 this represents | US$ 2,500,000 |

### *4.4. Gradual Approach to Landfill Improvement*

The purpose of the concept of step-by-step improvements over time is, initially, to improve disposal site operations and then later, improve disposal site design and engineering. This matches the gradual rise in sophistication of landfills in higher-income countries that has taken place over the past thirty years. An underlying rule of the 'gradual approach' is that whatever changes are possible at a disposal site, the resulting 'better landfill' should be an improvement on former practices.

### *4.5. Relevant Guidance*

Most guidance materials on landfilling are based on explanations of techniques and technologies suited to the conditions and regulations found in higher-income countries. They are often based on extremely high levels of protection of aquifers, incorporating a wide range of aesthetic issues, low noise, low gaseous emissions and high qualities of leachate treatment. Consequently, such guidance materials are not necessarily relevant to the requirements and capabilities of a municipality in a middle- or lower-income country.

The availability of good, relevant guidance, both written and on site, is an important prerequisite to launching a landfill improvement project. Many waste managers in middle- and lower-income countries are inexperienced in designing and operating improved landfills. To address this deficiency, the best guidance documents are those that assist waste managers who are confident enough to take a lead in changing their landfill operations.

### *4.6. Countering Risk Aversion*

In most municipalities, changes and improvements to the waste system bring uncertainty. Improvements to a landfill operation are a prime cause of uncertainty. Uncertainty that the improvements will not work and uncertainty whether or not the waste managers will be criticised, or worse, dismissed. Since no manager wants to be ridiculed or humiliated by the elected members or the media over an attempt to try something better, they are naturally cautious about starting. It is disappointing to observe that municipal leaders are too often quick to criticise public servants and slow to applaud their achievements. The effort and support involved in working with waste managers to overcome their aversion to the risk of trying something new should not be under-estimated. The successful implementation of a landfill improvement project depends upon it.

### *4.7. Co-operative Roles for Enforcement and Training*

Improvements to landfill operations, or any other waste management activity, cannot occur in a vacuum. Basic laws are necessary to empower municipalities to undertake collection and dispose of municipal wastes, as well as to provide powers to control abuse involving waste. Without some waste legislation it is difficult to motivate waste managers to change their practices. They can argue that if there is no legal requirement then they have no obligation make a change. This type of excuse has been used in some cities to avoid providing waste collection services to squatter settlements, since in law waste services only need to be provided for authorised dwellings. Similar arguments are sometimes applied to avoid closing down informal open dump sites. The absence of a law stating that only permitted (licensed) sites can be used for waste disposal means a municipality may have less power to stop them.

All improvements in a waste operation require learning new approaches or techniques, and gaining the confidence to keep them going. There is sometimes a 'knowledge gap' in a municipal waste department and managers may have genuine difficulty in envisaging how a proposed improvement will benefit their operations or the community.

Training, either through study visits or on-the-job, are the usual responses to close the knowledge gap. Until the knowledge gap is reduced, the chances of an improved landfill operation being run well and the improvement replicated are slim. Well thought-out and specific training is akin to an insurance policy for a landfill improvement project. As such, it is an important prerequisite to providing sustained improvements to land disposal.

## 5. Conclusions

It has been a long struggle for higher-income countries to achieve the standard of sanitary landfill they have come to expect. Depending on the precision of the comparison made, it is estimated that this process took one and a half generations (say thirty-five years). Waste managers elsewhere look, sometimes with envy, and sometimes with bemusement, at the complexity of the role expected from their higher-income counterparts. Often it is remarked that operating sanitary landfills is a ‘rich man’s pastime’. Whilst there is an economic link between the level of sophistication achievable and the level of finance available, it can be argued that waste managers elsewhere can still do much to adopt the fundamental approach to ‘controlling and isolating’ waste, even at the most basic disposal site.

For managers in middle- and lower-income countries, moving from a municipal culture of accepting open dumping as an inevitable fact of life to one where engineering improvements are encouraged and supported, is a road that still has to be travelled. Many places are only at the beginning and in spite of mass communication, it is difficult to see the thirty-five-year time scale dropping to between twenty and twenty-five years in all but the most fortunate countries who receive windfall incomes from the exploitation of their natural oil or gas resources. Consequently, the continuing role of professional waste organisations and international agencies in this field should be:

- to understand the fear of the waste manager, most likely of relatively low status in the municipality hierarchy, of trying something new and to tailor assistance to overcoming his or her fear;
- to encourage and support more waste managers to try out modest improvements in their landfill operations and then to build their confidence making further improvements in the future;
- to encourage municipalities not to forget waste disposal, and to urge them to increase the budgetary provision for better landfill;
- to recognise that the development of better landfills has to go through a sequential series of changes and that giant leaps in technological improvement are rarely successful; and
- to ensure that the assistance given is appropriate to the present stage of landfill development in each community.

Recently, the WHO has proposed several ways in which individuals and organisations from higher-income countries could work together with their counterparts elsewhere. The non-exhaustive list of options for those interested in the international aspects of waste management is reproduced below in the hope that it will stimulate even more innovative ideas (Rushbrook, 1996):

- managers could be released for short-term voluntary assistance (two, three, four or more weeks) in the field on defined projects;
- municipalities could include technical assistance to waste departments in their twinning programmes to towns outside western Europe;
- professional and academic institutions could twin with fledgling professional and academic bodies elsewhere to encourage their development, or even set up overseas branches;
- municipalities and waste operators could offer longer-term secondments of their personnel for three, six or twelve months and present it as an advantage in their career development;
- municipalities, institutions and even waste operators could offer equipment sponsorship, travel and study bursaries and even help with language training;

- municipalities, institutions, waste operators and independent bodies could provide technical waste management literature and underwrite regular subscriptions to waste journals;
- institutions could provide access to their certified training programmes for waste managers. Participation in Western training courses leading directly, or eventually, to a Western professional qualification or membership is particularly sought after;
- institutions could offer heavily-discounted membership subscriptions or fees to managers from middle- and lower-income countries;
- institutions, or the waste sector collectively, could establish a development fund to support two or three field projects in the Eastern European area and build up a long-term relation with the recipient cities and countries; and
- waste operators and municipalities could offer used but serviceable waste equipment to Eastern European towns as a temporary measure to overcome their shortage of resources.

## Author's Note

This article should be regarded as an anthology. It draws extensively upon previous papers published recently by the author. The relevant papers are listed below:

Rushbrook, P.E. (1998) Pre-requisites for successful implementation of landfill guidelines, *Proc. ISWA World Congress 1998*, Charlotte, NC, USA, 26-29 October 1998.

Rushbrook, P.E. (1998) The internationalisation of waste management, *Proc. IWM (Institute of Wastes Management, UK) Midlands Centenary Meeting*, Birmingham, UK, 14 September 1998, IWM, Northampton, UK.

Rushbrook, P.E. (1997) Getting from subsistence landfill to sophisticated landfill, *Proc. ISWA'97 World Conference*, Wellington, New Zealand, 29 September to 3 October 1997. Also published in (1999) *Waste Management & Research* **17 (1)**, 4-9.

Rushbrook, P.E. (1996) Achieving improved waste management: a programme to put theory into practice, presented at solid waste management workshops in Sarajevo and Banja Luka, Bosnia Herzegovina, June 1996 and April 1997 respectively.

## References

Diaz, L.F., Savage, G.M., Eggerth, L.L., and Golueke, C.G. (1996) *Solid Waste Management for Economically Developing Countries*, International Solid Waste Association (ISWA), Copenhagen, Denmark.

Government of South Africa (1994) *Minimum Requirements for Waste Disposal by Landfill*, First edition, Department of Water Affairs and Forestry, Pretoria, South Africa.

Rushbrook, P.E. (1996) Development assistance in waste management in Eastern Europe: waste organisations can do much to help, *Proc. 7th ISWA International Congress*, Pacifico Yokohama, Japan, 27 October to 1 November 1996.

Rushbrook, P.E. (1998) Editorial, *Waste Management & Research* **16 (5)**, 401-402.

Rushbrook, P.E., and Pugh, M.P. (1999) Solid waste landfills in middle- and low-income countries: a technical guide to planning, design and operation, Jointly produced by the WHO Regional Office for Europe, World Bank, Swiss Development Corporation (SDC), and Swiss Centre for Development Co-operation in Technology and Management (SKAT), *World Bank Technical Paper No. 426*, World Bank, Washington DC, USA.

## Disclaimer

This paper contains the personal opinions of the author and does not necessarily reflect the views of the World Health Organisation.

# WASTE MANAGEMENT: AN INDUSTRIAL POLICY POINT OF VIEW

O. LINHER
*European Commission, DG III*
*Wetstraat 200*
*B-1049 Brussels*
*BELGIUM*

**Summary**

This article describes the main principles of Community waste legislation with a particular emphasis on issues relevant from the point of view of industrial policy. It shows the merits and limitations of concepts such as the waste management hierarchy and producer responsibility. The main new instruments applicable to landfills and incinerators are discussed. An overview of instruments to encourage prevention, re-use and recycling is given.

## 1. Introduction

Within the European Commission, waste management is the primary responsibility of Directorate General XI (Environment). Since the Commission is a collective organ, other DG's also have units or officials who are supposed to guarantee consistency between the various policies. Since industry is one of the main implementors of waste management policies, DG III (Industry) has a particular interest in these issues.



*P. Nicolopoulou-Stamati et al. (eds.), Health Impacts of Waste Management Policies,* 57–62.

The basic Commission reference document with respect to waste management policy is the Community Strategy for Waste Management which was most recently reviewed in 1996 (COM(96) 399 final). This document outlines the main goal of a Community policy in this field (*'to achieve a high degree of environmental protection without distorting the functioning of the Internal Market with a view to promoting sustainable development'*; p. 1a), discusses basic concepts and gives an overview of the main instruments of waste policy.

## 2. Principles Underlying the EU Waste Policy

One of the basic concepts in waste management policy is the so-called 'hierarchy of waste management options'. As useful as this general rule is, it is subject to gross misunderstanding. As the Strategy states, the hierarchy is a basic rule that *'needs to be applied with a certain flexibility'* (p. 6). Prevention of waste shall be seen as a preferable option to recovery and final disposal of waste. Within the recovery option, preference should, in general, be given to material over energy recovery operations, where environmentally sound.

This rule needs to be seen in a wider context. Obviously, prevention cannot always prevail since waste is closely associated with life and economic activity. It is, however, the goal of Community policy to keep the levels of waste as low as possible and to reduce the impact of waste on the environment to a minimum. In this context, waste policy should however not be seen isolated from, but integrated into a policy that minimises the effect of a product throughout its whole life cycle, from production to use, and finally to its waste stage.

The preferences expressed in the hierarchy are based on the assumptions that the lower options entail externalities, i.e. that they cause pollution which is not truly reflected in the price of waste management. Concrete policies should therefore give incentives and regulations which favour the higher options. As a broad rule, this is a valuable guideline. This should, however, not hide the fact that the hierarchy is not a goal per se, especially not if the higher options result in more pollution.

It is frequently overlooked that waste management is not a choice between causing pollution or not but a choice between various forms of environmental impact, some of them more serious than others. It is a mistake to believe that recycling and re-use do not cause pollution. All recycling and re-use processes need energy and give rise to emissions. The aim of the legislator is therefore to find the optimal ways to encourage, promote and, if necessary, prescribe less environmentally damaging options at a minimum cost to society.

Another basic principle discussed in the Waste Management Strategy is the so-called 'producer responsibility'. The core of the concept is to involve the producer, financially and/or physically, in the waste management of his product, thus providing an incentive for environmentally friendly design. Again, this is a useful principle which should be used wherever positive results can be achieved. Once again, it is necessary to underline the limits of this concept which is in no way the solution to all waste management problems.

Producer responsibility works well in cases where the identification of the producer is easy and where the cost differences are sufficient to encourage an improvement in design. This is, however, not always the case. It should not be overlooked that the costs of such systems are not borne by the producers themselves but are usually passed on to the consumer. It is therefore necessary to create efficiency in such systems and avoid situations where costs are multiplied without a corresponding environmental benefit.

## 3. Instruments in the EU Waste Policy

Through the instruments for the implementation of waste management policy, the Commission pursues a strategy of high standards for waste treatment installations throughout the Community, in order to guarantee maximum environmental and health protection on the one hand, and to promote higher options in the waste management hierarchy on the other. Transboundary flows of wastes to cheaper, less efficient installations should be avoided through common standards. For disposal operations, the principles of proximity and self-sufficiency apply. At the same time, recovery operations should be encouraged by allowing trade with a minimum of administrative requirements (such trade has to follow the rules of the Community Waste Shipments Regulation 259/93).

After years of discussion, the adoption of a Directive on Landfills by the Council of Ministers is imminent. It foresees three classes of landfill, obligatory pre-treatment of wastes, reduction of biodegradable wastes going to landfill, prohibition of certain wastes in landfills (including waste tyres) and a transparent cost calculation (including aftercare for a minimum of thirty years). Through the implementation of this Directive, the environmental impact of landfills (*inter alia* leachates and methane emissions, disamenities for neighbouring population) will be reduced substantially. Precarious landfills, which are still widespread throughout the Community, will be eliminated.

The Commission has recently adopted a proposal for a Directive on Incineration of (non-hazardous) Waste. This directive will replace the existing Directives on Incineration of Municipal Waste and complement the existing Directive on Incineration of Hazardous Waste (94/67/EC). It will considerably strengthen the requirements for waste incinerators, including installations, previously not covered such as cement kilns and co-incineration power plants. The directive also prescribes energy recovery from incineration wherever feasible.

Among the pollutants addressed, an economic and scientific analysis (ETSU, 1996) stressed the importance of confronting the issue of particulate matter, partly created through secondary formation from $NO_x$ and $SO_2$. Emissions of dioxins and furans were evaluated as only of secondary importance in the concentrations realistically occurring in the vicinity of waste incinerators performing up to the existing standards. Nevertheless, the Community is addressing public concerns about dioxins and furans by setting the very strict standard of 0,1 ng/m$^3$. If all incinerators perform to this standard, this would mean a reduction in excess of 99 per cent relative to 1993/95 levels, making incinerators an almost negligible source of these substances. However, it is evident that even the existing standards are a long way from being implemented throughout the Community.

Along with standards for treatment installation, the Commission pursues a policy of actively encouraging the prevention, re-use and recycling of waste wherever this makes sense. Examples of such Directives are the Packaging and Packaging Waste Directive

(94/62/EC) and the Directive on Batteries and Accumulators (91/157/EEC). Current projects in this direction are the Commission Proposal for a Directive on End of Life Vehicles (COM(97) 358 final)[1] and the draft Proposal for a Directive on Waste from Electrical and Electronic Equipment. Finally, the Commission has issued a Communication on the Competitiveness of the Recycling Industries (COM(98) 463 final). On this basis, a Forum for Recycling is created with the aim of proposing options to further encourage recycling.

## 4. Conclusions

For the legislator, waste management poses a challenge to adopt effective strategies for the minimisation of the impact of waste in the context of the whole life cycle of products. As regards the health impacts of landfills and incineration, currently the biggest task for administrations is to ensure the effective implementation of existing EU rules as well as the future Landfill and Incineration Directives which are soon to be adopted. The elimination of improper installations alone will result in the reduction of the main effects of incinerators (particles, dioxins, etc.) and landfills (methane, uncontrolled leachates, etc.) to a fraction of current emissions. This should also prevent waste going to badly managed but cheap installations instead of properly equipped plants. Further reduction in emissions and linked health effects can be achieved through prevention at source, i.e. the prohibition in new products of substances which might have negative effects during their waste stage. Moreover, the re-use and recycling of waste can, to a certain extent, reduce environmental impacts leading to health effects. Generally speaking, however, it is necessary to carefully evaluate such options since there are substantial misconceptions about the real impact of certain substances. Equally, environmental pollution from re-use and recycling tends to be overlooked in the public discussion.

---

[1] Published in C337 of 07-11-1997, p. 3.

## References

ETSU (1996) Economic Evaluation of the Draft Incineration Directive, A report produced for the European Commission DG XI.

## Disclaimer

The opinions expressed in this article are those of the author only and do not necessarily reflect those of the European Commission.

# NATIONAL POLICY LINES ON WASTE MANAGEMENT

# THE EUROPEAN ENVIRONMENTAL BUREAU ON THE EUROPEAN COMMISSION'S PROPOSAL ON INCINERATION OF WASTE

D. SOTIROPOULOS-VARDAKA
*European Environmental Bureau*
*Bld. de Waterloo 34*
*B-1000 Brussels*
*BELGIUM*

## Summary

This article sets out the main objectives of the European Commission's Proposal for a Council Directive on Incineration of Waste (COM (1998) 558 final) as well as the comments and proposals made by the European Environmental Bureau.

The Directive aims at reducing the negative effects of waste incineration and co-incineration on the environment and human health.

The European Environmental Bureau (EEB) considers that the draft Directive misses the chance to introduce further incentives to avoid incineration of waste to the benefit of the re-use or recycling of waste, and estimates that the Emission Level Values (ELVs) are too high. Further, it is in disagreement with the absence of provisions regarding the environmental health-related surveillance of incinerators and deplores the fact that the draft falls short with regard to the promotion of the prevention of waste through raising public awareness and education, especially due to the of lack of a 'precautionary approach'.



*P. Nicolopoulou-Stamati et al. (eds.), Health Impacts of Waste Management Policies, 65–72.*

## 1. Introduction

The paper aims to give a short presentation of the position of the EEB on the proposal of the European Commission for a Directive on the incineration of waste.

It has to be recognised from the outset that the competence of the Union (and, indirectly, of the Commission as the initiator of legislation) in this respect is only complementary to that of the Member States. However, since the proposals of the European Commission give the basic guidelines to the Member States in relation to their relevant legislation, their significance should not be underestimated.

The incineration of waste is a subject of considerable public concern in the European Union. There are already 845 municipal waste incinerators in the EU and production of waste will continue to rise. It is widely recognised that whilst incineration of waste can form an important part of an integrated waste management system, strict controls are required to prevent adverse environmental effects.

## 2. The Proposal of the European Commission

In order to improve the protection of both the environment and public health, the European Commission is working on a proposal for a Directive on the incineration of waste. The aim of this Directive is to prevent or to reduce the negative effects of the incineration and co-incineration of waste on the environment, in particular air, soil, surface and groundwater pollution, and the resulting risks to human health, and to set up and maintain appropriate operating conditions and emission limit values for the incineration and co-incineration plants within the Community.

The Directive covers installations for the incineration and co-incineration of waste, (excluding hazardous and radioactive waste, wood and wood residues) and plants that treat less than 10 tonnes per year of non-municipal waste only. Member States shall adopt the laws, regulations and administrative provisions necessary to comply with this Directive no later than two years after its entry into force.

The key objectives of this proposal are:

- the setting of total emission limit values in order to substantially reduce emissions of several pollutants into the air, and control pollution of water and land in accordance with the Fifth Action Programme on the Environment;
- the provision of a coherent methodology for the regulation and operation of non-hazardous waste incineration and co-incineration to minimise the impact of both. Incineration and co-incineration will comply with the same 'Total Emission Values';
- the control and monitoring of air emissions from incineration plants for municipal waste. Continuous measurements for CO, total dust, TOC, HCl, $SO_2$, $NO_x$ and at least two measurements per year for heavy metals, dioxins and furans;
- the integration of the latest technological advances into EU legislation;
- the access to information and public participation in the permit procedure.

*Table 5.* The daily emission limit values (ELV) for both incineration and co-incineration suggested by the European Commission[2].

| Pollutants | European Commission's proposal (in $mg/m^3$) | Special case of cement kilns (in $mg/m^3$) |
|---|---|---|
| Dust | 10 | 50 |
| HCl | 10 | 10 |
| HF | 1 | 1 |
| $SO_2$ | 50 | 200 |
| $NO_x$ | 200 (>300MWth)<br>400 (<300MWth) | 800 |
| Cd + Ti | 0.05 | 0.05 |
| Hg | 0.05 | 0.05 |
| Sb, As, Pb, Cr, Co, Cu, Mn, Ni, V | 0.5 | 0.5 |
| Dioxins and furans | 0.1 *ng/m*$^3$ | 0.1 *ng/m*$^3$ |

[2] The difference between household waste incinerators and cement kilns in the provisions of the draft Directive is due to the fact that cement kilns can be, under certain conditions, a good substitute for incinerators because of the high temperatures they can reach, permitting the reduction of emissions of dioxins and furans. Since in the cement kilns waste can be incinerated ('co-incinerated') with other fossil fuels, the requirements on emissions differ.

## 3. The Position of European Environmental Bureau (EEB)

EEB clearly prefers the prevention, re-use and recycling of non-hazardous waste instead of incineration and landfill, but as incineration is a matter of fact in the EU, EEB welcomes the European Commission's proposal, as there is an urgent need for such an initiative, not only for health and environmental reasons, but also for economic rationales. The EEB especially appreciates the introduction of regulatory measures for the co-incineration of all types of waste, as well as the introduction of emission limit values for dioxins and furans.

It is true that waste incineration reduces the amount of waste going to landfill, but at the same time it produces additional pollutants released into the air and water. For this reason, the incineration of municipal waste must be realised within a very rigid framework, with strict standards, requiring Best Available Technologies and accurate limit values.

Therefore the proposed Directive should be improved in the following five ways:

1. Co-generation (production of heat and power) should be made mandatory with a minimum of 30 per cent capture of energy, for waste streams with high calorific value for both incineration and co-incineration plants, to avoid wasting energy.

2. The permitting procedure should include provisions to avoid overcapacities, even if waste prevention is implemented. Incineration is not considered by EEB as the preferred solution for the prevention of pollution from waste. Therefore, overcapacity in incinerators risks creating incentives for this method, to the detriment of re-use or recycling. Further, overcapacities can create distortions in the 'flow' of waste between countries and, therefore, in the functioning of the internal market.

3. Pre-treatment of waste going to incineration or co-incineration must be mandatory in order to avoid either the incineration of waste which is re-usable or recyclable, or the incineration of waste containing heavy metals, which may increase their emission into the atmosphere or the presence of very toxic residues. Therefore, every shipment of waste must contain a clear indication that the types of waste to be incinerated are not suitable for re-use or material recycling. Also substances that might cause highly

toxic residues or emissions should definitely not be incinerated (e.g. PVC, heavy metals).

4. Emission Limit Values (ELVs) have to be adapted to what is today applied as BAT in the leading Member States (ELVs for the Netherlands and Germany are at least five times lower than those proposed by the European Commission).

*Table 6.* Current ranges of Best Permitting Practice for waste incineration plants.

| **Pollutant** | **Commission's Proposal - ELVs (in mg/m³) DAV/HAAV[1]** | **Dutch ELVs[2] (in mg/m³) HAV[1]** | **German Best Permitting Practice[3] (in mg/m³) DAV/HAAV[1]** |
|---|---|---|---|
| Dust | 10/30 | 5 | 0.05-5/5-30 |
| C | 10/20 | - | 1-5 |
| HCl | 10 | 10 | 0.3-5 |
| HF1 | 1 | 1 | 0.05-0.5 |
| $SO_2$ | 50/200 | 40 | 1.3-15/25 |
| $NO_2$ | 200/400 | 70 | 40/200 |
| Cd+Ti | 0.05 | 0.05 | 0.0002-0.005 |
| Hg | 0.05 | 0.05 | 0.001-0.02 |
| Total Heavy Metals | 0.5 | 1 | 0.004-0.1 |
| Dioxins and Furans | 0.1 *ng/m³* | 0.1 *ng/m³* | 0.001-0.05 *ng/m³* |

[1]DAV: Daily Average Value / HAAV: Half-hourly Average Value.
[2]Comments of the Dutch NGO 'Stichting Afval en Milieu' on the waste incineration directive.
[3]Source: Koordinationsstelle Genehmigungsverfahren (KGV), Öko-Institut e.V.

The EEB suggests a technologically forward-looking policy, instead of a backward oriented one. This means that the introduction of ELVs for waste incineration and co-incineration plants should be dynamic: to introduce existing best national standards when the directive comes into force and move towards more ambitious standards 5 years later (e.g. in 2007). This is not the case in the current European Commissions Proposal: generally one can say that most proposed ELVs for waste incineration plants are ten times higher than permitted practice!

The European Commission justifies the suggested ELVs with the argument that they go beyond the limits of a cost-benefit analysis (CBA). (ETSU, 1996)

Methodologically the CBA applies the *damage cost approach.* This approach monetarises external effect in a selective number of cases, and only where damage already has occurred can losses be estimated properly.

There are several perception filters to this approach:
1. not all damage might be identified,
2. of the damage identified, not all of it can be quantified, and
3. of the damage quantified, not all of it can be valued as a given amount of money (monetarised).

There are also some uncertainties associated with the benefit-analysis, such as:
- chronic effects of long-term exposure to low doses of these chemicals on mortality rates,
- pollution effects on ecological resources,
- non-carcinogenic effects of heavy metals and dioxins,
- determination of threshold concentration, etc.

Furthermore, the World Health Organisation is very likely to lower the acceptable level of daily intake of dioxins. This will again have an impact on the 'benefits' of a dioxin reduction policy. There also seem to be some uncertainties on the cost side. The CBA only analyses organisational measures and end-of-pipe solutions, such as flue gas treatment. Cost-benefit analysis in general, perhaps, a degree of the scientific precision of the 'benefits' of a specific measure, which they cannot fulfil. The optimal level of pollution remains for the time being a theoretical construction of economists, but not an empirically valid concept. Therefore a positive CBA study - benefits exceed the costs - can only be used as an additional justification for strict standards. Negative CBA results are not necessarily a justification for non-action.

The *precautionary approach* deals with uncertainties. It deals with minimising the risks, where the exact costs and benefits are not known. The EEB therefore suggests formulating ELVs on the basis of Best Permitting Practice and not upon refutable economic evaluation studies.

5. A combined approach should be promoted, which would include emission limit values as well as air quality values, to avoid environmental deterioration and health problems in heavily polluted regions. In such areas, stringent Emissions Limit Values are not sufficient to prevent additional health problems from waste incineration. The EEB proposes to include a formulation similar to Art. 10 of the IPPC (Integrated Pollution and Control) Directive in the Waste Incineration Directive:

   *'Where an environmental quality standard requires stricter conditions than those achievable by the Emission Limit Values of this directive, additional measures shall in particular be required in the permit. No permit for a new plant can be delivered, if due to the plant the environmental quality standards should be exceeded.'*

## 4. Conclusions

Taking into account the well-known Lansink waste hierarchy, the EEB's policy is based on prevention, re-use and material recycling methods and not on waste incineration. This means that avoiding overcapacities in the planning of incineration plants, which are counterproductive to waste prevention, must be a political priority and therefore included somehow in the Directive. In the case of waste substances that can be re-used, recycled or biologically treated after a separate collection or mechanical separation, incineration should be avoided.

Since waste incineration is an increasing reality in the European Union, it has to be realised in **a very strict framework**, with strict standards requiring best available technology and accurate limit values. The proposed emission limits in the Commission's proposal do not reflect the available techniques. They are lower than the ELVs of some leading Member States. The EEB believes that more improvements are feasible and would lead to greater public acceptance of incineration plants.

Furthermore, EEB believes that systematic 'environmental health surveillance' is needed at waste incineration and landfill sites that cause public or scientific concern. Surveillance should make use of the registers of congenital abnormality, include assessment of human exposure to chemicals, and encourage regular communication between departments with health and environmental responsibilities.

However, one should not forget that the main way to minimise health or environmental risks is the waste prevention policy. There are many instruments and strategies for such a policy, but one of the most important aims is to change the public perception on sustainable consumption and waste prevention through information campaigns and participation in debates (along with other NGOs, environmentally oriented consumer federations, local and national authorities, doctors, teachers, students, and schools). If people are made aware of the waste problem, they can be motivated to adopt common preventative measures that will have positive effects on both their health and the environment.

## References

ETSU (1996) Economic evaluation of the draft incineration directive, a report produced for the European Commission DGXI, Contract number B4 3040/95/001047/ MAR/B1.

EC (1996) The IPPC Council Directive: Integrated Pollution Prevention and Control (1996/6/EC).

# HOUSEHOLD WASTE MANAGEMENT IN THE FLEMISH REGION OF BELGIUM

L. VAN GRIMBERGEN
*Flemish Public Waste Agency*
*(Openbare Vlaamse Afvalstoffenmaatschappij)*
*Kan. de Deckerstraat 22-26*
*B-2800 Mechelen*
*BELGIUM*

**Summary**

The Flemish region, in northern Belgium, has six million inhabitants, which is four hundred and thirty-seven inhabitants per square kilometre.

The key objective laid down in the waste prevention and waste management decree of 2 July 1981 is to protect human health and the environment from the harmful effects of waste and to avoid the wastage of raw materials and energy. This is reflected in a waste management strategy ranging from the prevention of waste through recovery, by re-use of products, recycling material, energy recovery for use as fuel and disposal of waste by incineration with energy recovery and landfill.

In 1997, Flemish municipalities collected 528 kg of household waste per inhabitant. Municipal waste collection services reach the entire population with door to door collections and collections at container parks. Separately collected household waste fractions are brought to authorised re-use or recovery installations. Vegetable, fruit and garden waste and green waste are composted. Incineration plants for combustible



*P. Nicolopoulou-Stamati et al. (eds.), Health Impacts of Waste Management Policies,* 73–88.

household waste and similar industrial waste have been modified to meet the most stringent EU standards and emission limit values for incineration of hazardous waste. All incinerators have energy recovery systems in operation. Non-recyclable and non-combustible household waste that is pre-treated and fulfils acceptance criteria goes to well-equipped landfills. Ecotaxes have been introduced on consumer goods. Levies have been put on incineration and landfill of waste. Producers and importers have take-back obligations regarding end of life consumer goods. A ban on landfilling and incineration of separately collected waste fractions as well as of mixed household waste has been implemented.

## 1. Introduction

The population of Belgium is ten million, and there are three hundred and twenty-three inhabitants per square kilometre. Belgium is a federal state with three regions:

- Flemish region
- Brussels capital region
- Walloon region

There are nearly six million inhabitants in the Flemish region. It is very densely populated with four hundred and thirty-seven inhabitants per square kilometre. The Flemish region contains three hundred and eight municipalities. Antwerp and Ghent are the largest cities. They are parts of conurbations of at least one million inhabitants. The country is further characterised by a wide scattering of quasi-urban settlements on rural land.

The governmental structure of Belgium is rather complex. The laws on the reform of the Belgian State transferred the competencies concerning the environment to the regions. Waste management also became an environmental competence of the regions. One major exception is the federal competence on nuclear waste. For the Flemish region, the Flemish Public Waste Agency, OVAM, was created on 1 October 1981. Its main tasks are the monitoring and implementation of waste prevention and waste management and the remediation of contaminated soil. It is a civil service with two hundred and sixty employees.

Except for the OVAM itself, a specific environmental inspection service of the ministry of the Flemish government manages the enforcement of environmental legislation, including waste legislation. The federal police, customs and judicial services are engaged by their general competencies in the enforcement of waste legislation. On a municipal level, environmental officials have local competencies on environmental issues.

## 2. Flanders' Environmental and Waste Legislation

Environmental legislation in the Flemish region was the subject of large debate for more than 10 years. An inter-university commission prepared a series of draft decrees on environmental issues (Interuniversitaire Commissie tot Herziening van het Milieurecht in het Vlaamse Gewest, 1985). Several decrees have since been adopted by the Flemish government.

The framework of the Flemish waste prevention and waste management legislation is detailed in the decree of 2 July 1981. Since the European directive 75/442 was amended by directive 91/156, the Flemish decree has also been amended by the decree of 20 April 1994. From 1981 to the present day several additional regulations have been approved by the Flemish parliament. The most recent regulation on waste was decided upon by the Flemish government on 17 December 1997. It consists of the amalgamation of previous decisions on waste regulation which were slightly amended, as well as of several new issues.

Closely related to waste management is the issue of contaminated land policy. Measures applicable to the investigation and clean-up of contaminated sites were included in the decree of 2 July 1981, until the decree of 22 February 1995 on soil clean-up was adopted. On 5 March 1996, the Flemish government adopted the necessary application measures.

The decree on the environmental permit of 28 June 1985 deals with the procedural aspects for those permits and is the legal basis for adopting general and sectoral environmental rules.

A decree on environmental agreements was enacted on 15 June 1994. Voluntary agreements were signed between the Flemish government and the appropriate industries concerning:

- batteries,
- end of life vehicles,
- discarded medicines.

The decree of 5 April 1995 on general aspects concerning environmental policy includes the set-up of a general environmental management plan. The first general environmental management plan covers the period of 1997-2001 (Vlaamse Regering, 1997). In Chapter 7, it covers the framework for waste management planning. The same decree requires a biennial environmental report. It was first published in 1994 (Verbruggen, 1994; Verbruggen, 1998). It contains the description, analysis and evaluation of the existing environmental situation, including a chapter on waste management.

Every year, an environmental action programme is established by the Flemish government in order to implement the management plan. To achieve certain goals, other sectoral plans can be drawn up. In this regard, a recent management plan on household waste was adopted. In addition, for VFG (vegetable, fruit and garden waste) and for construction and demolition waste, two management plans came into force.

## 3. Key Objectives

The key objective laid down in the waste decree is to protect human health and the environment from the harmful effects of waste and to avoid the waste of raw materials and energy. This is reflected in our waste management strategy, ranging from the prevention of waste to recovery, with the re-use of products, recycling of materials and energy recovery for use as fuel, and disposal of waste by incineration with energy recovery (in exceptional cases, incineration without energy recovery can be appropriate) and landfill. (OECD, 1998)

# 4. Prevention and Management of Household Waste

## 4.1. Generation

Household waste includes waste produced by private households and other waste collected by municipalities, i.e. waste from very small enterprises similar to household waste, that is allowed by local municipalities to be treated together with household waste; street waste, and public market waste collected by the municipalities.

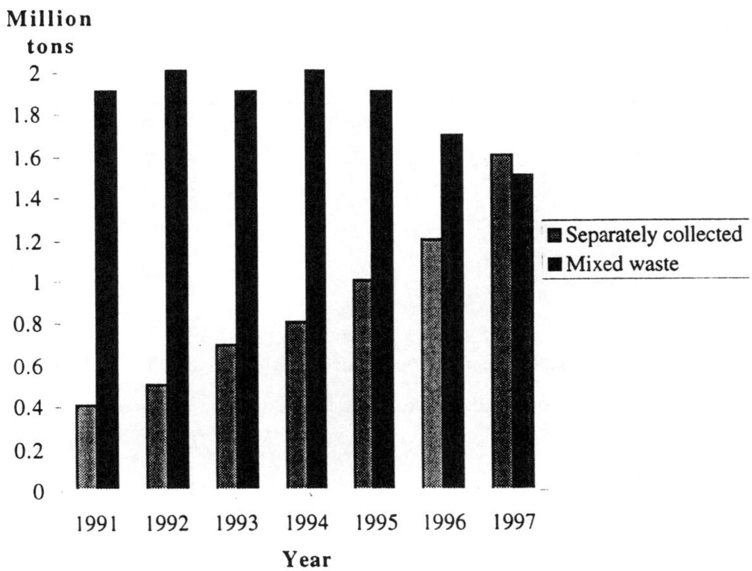


*Figure 3.* Household waste collection in Flanders.

In 1997, Flemish municipalities collected 3,115,013 tons of household waste (528 kg per inhabitant) (OVAM, 1997b). Municipal waste generation is still rising, although there was a slight indication of stabilisation before 1997. As Figure 3 shows, in the last decade the collection of household waste increased from 2.3 million tons in 1991 to 3.1 million tons in 1997 (Figure 3. Total sum of separately collected waste plus mixed waste). During the same period there was a noticeable shift in collection systems. Systematic action and sensitising of the public and local authorities resulted in a year-on-year increase of separately collected fractions. This separate collection is a first step towards optimising the treatment of waste, more specifically with respect to the recovery and recycling of materials. The public at large and local authorities showed willingness to co-operate for the sake of better waste management.

Actions and sensitising were not sufficient to provoke a decrease in collected quantities. Up to now, waste prevention has been insufficient and too localised for global effects on the production of household waste to be felt. Manufacturers of goods have to be made more responsible for the products they commercialise and for the waste yielded after consumption. The impact of waste management policy on ecodesign and cleaner production has been insufficient until now.

*Table 7.* Composition of household waste in Flanders (data for 1996).

| | |
|---|---|
| VFG waste (vegetables, fruit, garden) | 35.9 % |
| Paper and cardboard | 16.8 % |
| Glass | 5.5 % |
| Metals | 3.2 % |
| Textiles | 1.1 % |
| Plastics | 4.0 % |
| SHW (small scale hazardous waste) | 0.7 % |
| Construction and demolition waste | 13.0 % |
| Wood | 0.8 % |
| Other bulky waste | 11.0 % |
| Street and market waste | 2.6 % |
| Others | 5.4 % |
| Total | 100 % |

With regard to the overall composition of collected household waste, Table 7 provides the figures for 1996 on a weight basis. It should be noticed that more than one third of collected household waste by weight is in fact VFG waste. The volume of packaging waste (paper and cardboard, plastics, metals, glass) is by far the largest fraction. Apart from packaging waste, paper in household waste mainly consists of newspapers, magazines and advertising leaflets. The household waste-collecting systems which collect construction and demolition waste, collect only a very small part (<10 per cent) of the total supply of construction and demolition waste in the Flemish region. (OVAM, 1997a)

### *4.2. Collection*

By decree, municipalities have to collect all household waste in their municipality on a regular basis. Municipalities also have to maintain the cleanliness of streets and markets. To achieve this, most municipalities (with three exceptions) have constituted intermunicipal associations through which the collection and treatment of household waste reach the entire population. Several methods are used for collection, including door-to-door collections and collection at 'container parks'. Every municipality has one or more well-equipped sites where containers are placed to separately receive different fractions of household waste.

By the end of 1996, two hundred and seventy-nine container parks were available, serving 90 per cent of the population. This number is still increasing. Municipalities may obtain financial aid for the setting up of container parks. According to the household waste management plan, different collection modes, as shown in Table 8, are to be put in place.

*Table 8.* Household waste collection modes.

| Door-to-door | Container park |
|---|---|
| Mixed household waste | Green waste |
| Vegetable/ fruit/ garden waste | Glass |
| Packaging waste | Plastics |
| Bulky waste | Metals |
| | Wood |
| | Textiles |
| | Construction and demolition waste |
| | Small scale hazardous waste |

Glass is mainly collected via communal recycling bins placed on the street. Special attention is paid to small-scale hazardous waste, due to the danger to the environment and public health. Specialised collection systems have been elaborated and specialised sensitising education was needed to eliminate as much small-scale hazardous waste as possible from mixed waste. Collectors of small-scale hazardous waste need special permits, imposing a series of specific conditions for collection tools and personnel.

Separate collection has been shown to be the strongest guarantee of efficient recycling. That is the reason why we chose to push this separate collection as far as possible for the recycling of raw materials.

*Table 9.* Separately collected amounts of household waste in Flanders (in tons x 1000).

| | 1996 | 1997 | Increase |
|---|---|---|---|
| Vegetable/ fruit/ garden waste | 428 | 614 | 43 % |
| Paper and cardboard | 260 | 322 | 24 % |
| Glass | 120 | 131 | 9 % |
| Metals | 43 | 53 | 23 % |
| Textiles | 5 | 9 | 80 % |
| Plastics | 17 | 25 | 47 % |
| Construction and demolition waste | 330 | 380 | 15 % |
| Wood | 23 | 36 | 56 % |
| Others | 12 | 12 | 0 % |

Separated collection of several fractions of household waste is increasing yearly. In 1991, a separately collected amount of 0.4 million tons was reached. In 1997, 1.6 million tons of fractions of household waste were separately collected and this marked the first year in which the separately collected amount exceeded the mixed part. The amount of separately collected waste per capita increased from 74 kg in 1991 to 269 kg in 1997. Table 9 details separately collected household waste in 1996 and 1997. The collection of VFG waste is increasing considerably, because a larger part of the public is being reached. Paper and cardboard and glass have been collected separately for a much longer period. The percentage of recovery is now up to 80 per cent. The absolute increase of collected waste paper is a consequence of the increased production of waste paper. There are very few textiles in household waste collection. Separate collection systems and the re-use and recycling of textiles have been in operation for a very long time. The bulk of plastics in household waste is packaging waste. The separate collection of plastic, metal and other light-weight beverage packaging is increasing, and this is particularly due to the management policy which has put targets in place for re-use and recovery.

## 5. Recovery

### *5.1. Material Re-Use and Recycling*

Separately collected household waste fractions are first brought to sorting installations and then to authorised recovery installations. Sorted fractions can go different ways.

Re-use of products or materials is the first option. Second-hand shops for clothing, furniture, electric and electronic equipment are encouraged. Workshops for the repair of used appliances receive aid from the Flemish government in their starting-up period. Dismantling equipment to save spare parts is another way to re-use products.

A second option is to recycle materials. Sorted paper and cardboard, sorted ferrous and non-ferrous metals go to appropriate recycling plants. Plastics are sorted, washed, remelted and extruded to be used as secondary raw materials. Textiles are also recycled to a very large extent. There is a separate collection for batteries. In shops, schools and factories, one can find boxes to collect used batteries. Good results are especially obtained with school collections. After sorting, some batteries go for metal recycling, others are treated as hazardous waste. Building and demolition waste is treated in crushing and sieving plants to form new secondary raw materials that are used for foundations instead of sand or gravel.

Although more and more new initiatives are being taken and new recycling plants are being built, the sale of recycled products and secondary raw materials continues to be a very difficult market to control. Competition between virgin materials and recycled materials is very high.

### *5.2. Composting*

Vegetable, fruit and garden waste are composted. Special attention and special publicity is given to home composting. This means that people compost their own compostable fraction (VFG). Two goals are achieved in this way. Apart from diminishing the amount of waste to be collected, good compost for the garden is created. To stimulate home composting, financial aid is given for the purchase of a compost bin. Composting experts teach people how to properly compost.

However, the majority of the generated VFG is collected and composted in eighteen composting plants. There is currently an important lack of capacity. Two major systems are used. The aerobic composting system is the most frequently used one. Too often it gives off a bad smell, especially in summer periods although large biofilters are installed. That is the reason why the use of plastic collection bags should be avoided. The anaerobic composting system generates methane and is used in one plant on a wide scale. Electricity is produced from methane. In some plants, only green garden waste is composted. The quality of the compost is continuously controlled. A quality label is given.

## 6. Disposal

Although various efforts are made and continue to be made for the prevention and recovery of household waste, half of the collected household waste still has to be disposed of, and must be incinerated or landfilled. The development in the disposal of household waste is shown in Figure 4. A recent large decrease in the amounts going to landfills is mostly a result of the improved separate collection of VFG waste and its recovery.

### *6.1. Incineration*

At this moment, eleven incineration plants for combustible household waste and similar industrial waste are operating. Older units have been closed down in recent years and new projects have been announced, although there is strong opposition from the public, due to a fear of damage to the environment and human health. The scale of the recently built units and the projected units range from between 150,000 and 200,000 tons per year. The older units have capacities of between 40,000 t and 100,000 t.

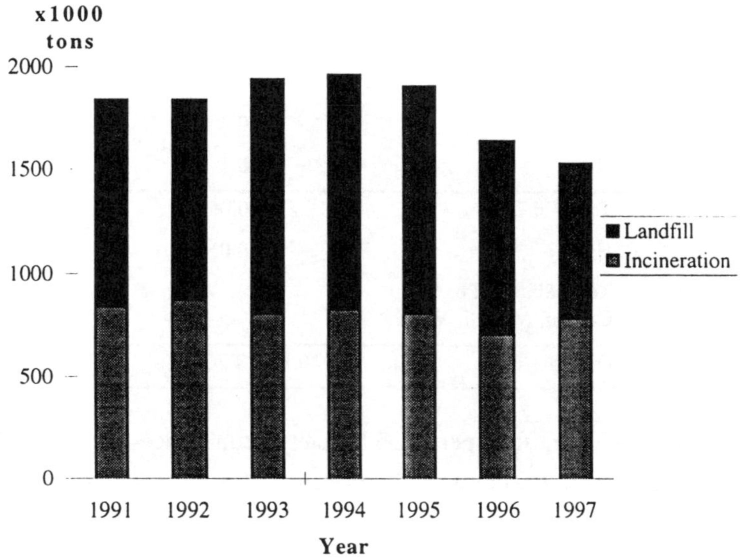


*Figure 4.* Disposal of household waste.

All units have been modified to meet the most stringent EU standards for incineration of hazardous waste. In Flemish legislation there is no longer a distinction in emission limit values between incineration of hazardous and non-hazardous waste. Table 10 provides air emission limit values for all incineration plants.

For dioxin the limit value is set at 0.1 ng TEQ/m$^3$. All incinerators in operation meet the required emission limit values. The results obtained are even better than legal levels.

In a first phase, improvements were carried out on the operation of the incineration process itself and on the operation of the flue gas treatment, mainly on the dust collection system. The subsequent phase was the addition of a dioxin capture system, usually activated carbon or lignite, combined with a filtering device. Continuous measurements of HCl, CO and dust are carried out. Heavy metals are measured at least twice a year. Continuous sampling of dioxin is imposed and an analysis is made every two weeks.

*Table 10.* Air emission limit values.

| | **Daily average values ($mg/m^3$)** |
|---|---|
| Total dust | 10 |
| TOC | 10 |
| HCl | 10 |
| $SO_2$ | 50 |
| $NO_x$ | 400 |
| Total Cd, TI | 0.05 |
| Hg | 0.05 |
| Total Sb, As, Pb, Cr, Co, Cu, Mn, Ni, V, Sn | 0.5 |
| Dioxin | 0.1 ng TEQ/$m^3$ |

Furthermore, incineration must be performed, in all circumstances, at a temperature of at least 850°C lasting at least 2 seconds in the presence of at least 6 per cent oxygen. As a consequence, all incinerators have to be equipped with support burners which have to operate automatically as soon as the temperature drops below 850°C. All incinerators have energy recovery systems in operation.

### *6.2. Landfill*

In the treatment of household waste, landfill is the very last option, after all other management methods designed for valorisation have been exhausted. This means that only non-recyclable and non-combustible household waste that is pre-treated can go to well equipped landfills. Acceptance criteria for waste in a landfill are fixed.

The installation and exploitation of a landfill must comply with several conditions. To protect soil and water, it is necessary to have a geological barrier consisting of a mineral layer with permeability requirements of $K \leq 1.0 \times 10^{-9}$ m/s and thickness requirements of at least 3 m on the bottom and at the sides of the landfill. In addition to the geological barrier, an artificial sealing liner of 2.5 mm HDPE or an equivalent has to be put into place between appropriate protection layers. Between the geological barrier and the artificial sealing liner a control drain is installed. On top of the artificial sealing liner a leachate collection system must be added. Leachate and surface water must be collected and treated in a wastewater treatment plant.

To protect groundwater, a number of measuring points have to be constructed. Sampling and analysis must take place on a regular basis. Landfilled waste is daily compacted to ensure stability of waste mass and is covered by a more inert layer to prevent emissions of odours and dust, sweep waste, birds and vermin and fires on the landfill.

Figure 4 shows the amounts of landfilled household waste from 1991 to 1997. After an increase in the first half of the nineties, a significant decrease is shown in 1996 and 1997. Since July the 1st 1998 there has been a ban on the disposal of mixed household waste. At this moment there is nevertheless no sufficient operational treatment capacity for the valorisation of all the recyclable and combustible waste. This means that some recyclable and combustible household waste is still collected as mixed waste and is sent to landfills, which constitutes an infringement of the rule.

Only twelve landfills for non-hazardous waste are in use. Four have a remaining capacity of 1 million $m^3$ or more. The others have remaining capacities ranging between 40,000 $m^3$ and 500,000 $m^3$. Due to strong local opposition, no new landfill sites will be allowed, and only an extension of existing landfills is possible. A landfill is considered closed if the required impermeable surface sealing layers and topsoil cover have been achieved on top of the landfill.

On biologically active landfills, a gas drainage layer is required. After landfill closure, an aftercare phase of at least ten years or more is necessary and required for monitoring and control.

## 7. Incentives and Requirements

A modern waste management strategy necessitates a mix of instruments.

### *7.1. Financial Instruments are Set Up*

The federal state introduced ecotaxes on certain consumer goods. Tax exemption applies if goods are taken back in a precautionary system. Levies are put on incineration of waste and on landfill of waste. Levies on incineration and landfill are set at such a level that the total cost for recovery is lower than the total cost for incineration and the latter still remains lower than the one for landfill. Prices without VAT for the incineration of household waste in incinerators equipped with flue gas treatment and energy recovery range from 52 Euros/ton to 70 Euros/ton with an additional levy of 6 Euros/ton. Prices for landfill of household waste are about 40 Euros/ton with an additional levy of 40 Euros/ton.

### *7.2. Producers Responsibility*

Take-back and acceptance obligations of consumer goods by producers, traders and importers have come into force. Producers and importers are responsible for recovery or disposal of end of life consumer goods, including waste or end of life printed paper, batteries, vehicles, tyres, electrical and electronic equipment and packaging. Producers and importers must accept end of life consumer goods with every purchase of a new product, from 1 July 2004, or even without the purchase of a new product. For printed paper containing publicity, and for batteries, the latter came into force in 1999. To achieve this, a voluntary agreement between representatives of producers and importers and the Flemish government may be signed, as was already done for batteries and end of life vehicles. Packaging waste has to be taken back by those responsible for the packaging, in line with the European packaging directive. Targets are set for collection and recovery of packaging waste.

### *7.3. Ban on Disposal*

Separate collection of paper and cardboard, glass, small-scale chemical waste and bulky waste from households is required. To make sure a higher degree of recovery is achieved, a ban on landfilling and on incineration came into force on 1 July 1998. As of 1 July 1998, separately collected paper and cardboard, greenwaste, VFG-waste, packaging waste of glass, metal, plastic and other packaging of drinks were no longer allowed on landfills and are no longer allowed for incineration as of 1 July 2000. Moreover, it was also forbidden to landfill mixed household waste as of 1 July 1998, and to incinerate it from 1 July 2000.

## 8. Conclusions

During the last decade, the waste management approach in the Flemish region, and especially as far as household waste is concerned, has been subject to profound change. The policy shifted from landfilling and incinerating to prevention and recycling. Sensitising the general public and local authorities is absolutely vital for the implementation of this management policy. The public and local authorities have shown a willingness to co-operate with this policy.

The first signs are appearing, that the increase in per capita municipal waste generation may have reached a maximum. Up to now, measures for the prevention of the generation of waste have had no effect whatsoever on the collected quantities of household waste. Efforts to reduce waste at source must be extended. The responsibilities of manufacturers must also be extended. Ecodesign and cleaner production should also be enforced to limit the generation of waste so as to prevent its harmful effects. This can be achieved by the introduction of less toxic materials in new products. Integration of product policy and waste management policy will be the challenge for the next decade.

The re-use and recycling of materials is widespread. Recycling targets have been met for some types of materials. Markets for recycled products are nevertheless difficult to control and will have to be encouraged by policy measures. Incineration and landfilling of non-recyclable waste in well-equipped installations are still an option. However, siting new landfills and incineration plants meets strong local opposition. The control and monitoring of incineration plants and landfills will have to improve to avoid adverse effects on the environment and human health.

## References


Interuniversitaire Commissie tot Herziening van het Milieurecht in het Vlaamse Gewest (1995) *Voorontwerp Decreet Milieubeid*, Die Keure, Brugge. (in Dutch)

OECD (1998) *Environmental Performance Review Belgium*, Paris.

OVAM (1997a) *Bedrijfsafvalstoffen, Extrapolatie van Meldingsgegevens*, Mechelen, Belgium. (in Dutch)

OVAM (1997b) *Uitvoeringsplan Huishoudelijke Afvalstoffen 1997-2001*, Mechelen, Belgium. (in Dutch)

Verbruggen, A. (ed.) (1994) *Leren om te Keren, Milieu- en Natuurrapport Vlaanderen*, Garant, Leuven-Apeldoorn. (in Dutch)

Verbruggen, A. (ed.) (1998) *Mira-T 1998, Milieu- en Natuurrapport Vlaanderen*, Garant, Leuven-Apeldoorn. (in Dutch)

Vlaamse Regering (1997) *Mina-plan 2, Het Vlaamse Milieubeleidsplan 1997-2001*, Aminal, Brussels. (in Dutch)

# WASTE-TO-ENERGY AND WASTE MANAGEMENT: AUSTRIAN AND EU POLICY LINES

*Objectives, Principles, Good Practice of the State of the Art and Current Issues*

R.L. LINDBAUER
*AE Energietechnik*
*P.O.B. 1004*
*A-8021 Graz*
*AUSTRIA*

## Summary

The objectives and principles of integrated waste management are very similar in Austria and the European Union. Introduction of these objectives and principles meant, for Europe, a technological revolution of integrated waste management to meet the demands of the precautionary principle: implementation of preventive or reduction schemes; initiation of material recycling and re-use; revamping and building a new generation of improved dedicated waste incinerators for that fraction of the waste which cannot be prevented, re-used or recycled. These improved dedicated waste incinerators have to comply with the demands of low emission limits. Equally, they can be considered to act as sinks for hazardous substances rather than as diffuse sources of pollution such as landfills for untreated waste.

The precautionary principle and subsequent performance standards - for obvious reasons of health care and environmental protection - must also apply to industrial co-incineration due to increased probability of hazardous contents in 'secondary products'.



*P. Nicolopoulou-Stamati et al. (eds.), Health Impacts of Waste Management Policies,* 89–105.

The proposed solution is embodied in the concept of 'material flow analysis'. This entails that incineration plants act as 'sinks' for hazardous substances in waste: i.e. they destroy organic components by heat and concentrate hazardous inorganic substances from the original waste rather than disseminating them in a diffuse way. Emission standards for this type of incinerator have been set by pro-active authorities, based upon the 'precautionary principle', in such a way that immission limits in the neighbourhood of these plants are not exceeded under any meteorological instances. Continuous emissions-monitoring of a number of inorganic and organic gases, such as HCl, SO, CO, TOC, dust and others, guarantee a safe, permanent operation. Co-incineration processes or plants using waste derived or secondary fuels should, of course, adhere to the same continuous monitoring scheme as well as to equal standards of emission limits.

## 1. Introduction

The practice of landfilling untreated waste which, especially in southern countries, has a high tendency to self-ignite, is no longer acceptable. There is no compliance with emission criteria aiming at the safeguarding of human health or the protection of the environment. Uncontrolled waste disposal leads to diffuse pollution on an unpredictable time-scale without knowledge of future costs for remedial actions.

The ASPIS programme aims at raising awareness and stimulating education on environmental health issues. In particular this seminar raises consciousness and awareness of the European Directives concerning the proper handling of waste. They include policy *objectives* and *principles* (EU Waste Framework Directive 75/442/EEC as amended by 91/156EEC). Among them is the *'essential objective of all provisions relating to waste disposal'* being *'...the protection of human health and the environment against harmful effects...'*

This objective must be reached by a hierarchical set of *principles:*
Prevention of waste is the first principle in this hierarchy. Obviously, waste which is not generated needs no disposal. Whether this principle leads to cleaner production and cleaner products is debatable. In this context, re-use and recycling which allow for the maximum recovery of products, is the sole option. It is our understanding that - since all products become waste at some time - we have to recover whatever of our products have finally become waste after their useful life cycle. If material recovery (re-use, recycling) is not possible for ecological or economic draw-backs, energy recovery is the preferred option. This re-use, recycling option is the second principle in a waste management strategy.

The third principle, a safe disposal of waste, can only be reached by conscious and conscientious treatment of waste with special attention paid to possible hazardous constituents. This means that treatment has to provide a final sink for the hazardous contents so that it can be stored safely and isolated from the biosphere (this means no harmful leachates, no toxic gases). The preferential option is to do this by thermal treatment and energy recovery; 'Waste-to-energy' as recovery and treatment option alike provides the final sink for harmful substances after their life cycle in products.

Waste incinerators are important for the objective of the third principle to be achieved: they are the only option available to deal with unpreventable and unrecoverable waste. This objective has not changed since they were initially introduced. The first waste incinerator on the continent, in Hamburg, Germany, was installed and inaugurated in 1895, more than one hundred years ago. This incinerator (Figure 5) was set up after the cholera epidemic in 1892 which originated from the Hamburg landfill. What has changed during the last century is the technical and technological practice, and performance of waste incineration, especially during the last 10 to 15 years. In particular, emission limits introduced by national and European regulations now assure low emission and immission values.[3]

---

[3] Editorial footnote: A major point to make is that the nature of the waste has changed since 1892. it now contains much higher levels of man-made (halogenated) plastics and heavy metals.

# ELEKTRIZITÄT AUS KEHRICHT

VON

ETIENNE DE FODOR

K. UNG. HOFRAT

GENERALDIREKTOR DER BUDAPESTER ALLGEMEINEN ELEKTRIZITÄTS-GESELLSCHAFT

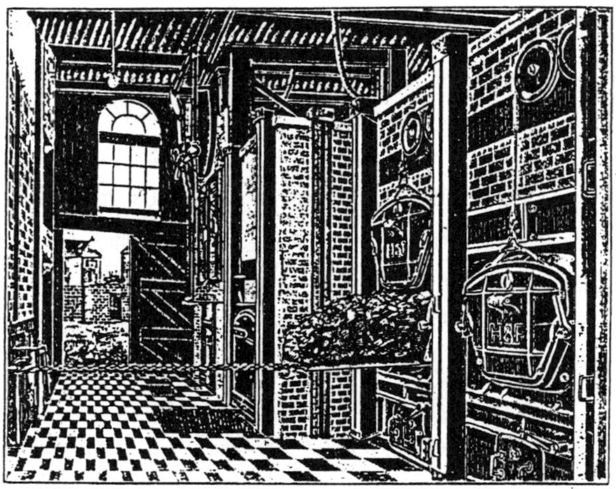

MIT 170 ORIGINAL-ABBILDUNGEN

BUDAPEST, 1911.

K. U. K. HOFBUCHHANDLUNG VON JULIUS BENKÖ

(V., DOROTTYA-UTCZA 2)

*Figure 5.* Cover page of De Fodor's book on waste incineration and electricity generation which was published at the beginning of the 20th century (De Fodor, 1911).

## 2. The Unstated Generally Valid Definition of Waste

Defining waste is not easy. The EU-Commission states (EU COM (96) 399):

> *'...discussion on the distinction between waste and goods has been going on for almost twenty years - no satisfactory objective definition has yet been found to determine when a material becomes waste and when waste become goods again...'*

In a report by IPTS (Bontoux and Leone, 1997) the authors are even more critical:

> *'...the waste definition from the Framework Directive on Waste is both so broad and imprecise that it leaves a lot of room for interpretation...'*
> *'...in the context of OECD decisions, the term* "disposal" *used to define* "waste" *includes its consignment to a recovery operation...'* whereas *'...the notion of discarding appears to be the decisive factor in determining whether a material is a waste ...'*

### *2.1. The Definition of Waste and the Treatment of Waste*

Over a 20-year period waste management has been the subject of more than 40 acts of legislation in the European Union. Nevertheless, the introduction of a Common Strategy for Waste Management - one of the key sectors identified by the Fifth Action Programme on the Environment to achieve sustainable development - was a Herculean task due to the lack of an agreed definition of waste or treatment of waste.

Not unexpectedly, the member states also face this problem. This explains, for example, why waste statistics in various countries show incongruent data. Professionals in the field have to deal with a regulatory framework which is dense and often difficult to interpret, flooded by varied and inconsistent 'lists of wastes' established by different organisations and/or member states. As a result, important discrepancies exist in Europe with respect to converting EU Directives into national law. For this latter phenomenon there are at least three reasons:

- many countries have been establishing their own policy and legislation to deal with waste for years. These historical differences among the member states complicate the incorporation of the EU Directives into the national/federal regulation;
- different sets of values, procedures, responsibilities, and institutions, exist in the member states as a result of the different waste policies in the past, and of geographical conditions, and practices;
- a weakly-defined, commonly accepted waste terminology, often mistaking the goal with the instruments, or the objectives with the principles.

### *2.2. A 'Leaky' Integrated Waste Management*

Integrated waste management was set up during the last 10 years in most European countries. The general objective of this policy is *'protect human well-being and the natural environment'*. Integrated waste management prefers waste prevention to material and energy recovery. Only the remaining fraction which cannot be prevented or recovered will be disposed of. These principles are counteracted in different ways: systemic or semantic evasion; unequal use of standards; control-wise impractical, exchangeable/varied lists of wastes; escape routes with technical dress-up features opening up new environmental - intermediate compartments such as secondary products or fuels, apart from the ones already known (air, water, soil) etc.

The discussion on waste is also hampered by the changing designation of waste; what is waste at a particular moment or place, can be a resource at another time or location.

Figures 6 and 7 illustrate possible results of these inconsistencies. Figure 6 shows the state of 'waste disposal' prior to 'integrated waste management' ('pre-1990') where the product and waste stream is 'throughput' oriented. Figure 7 shows the situation after the introduction of 'prevention' and 're-use/recycling' schemes. This leads to smaller quantities of waste to be disposed/landfilled. But this also (unintentionally) results in materials leaving their waste status, to be re-used as products.

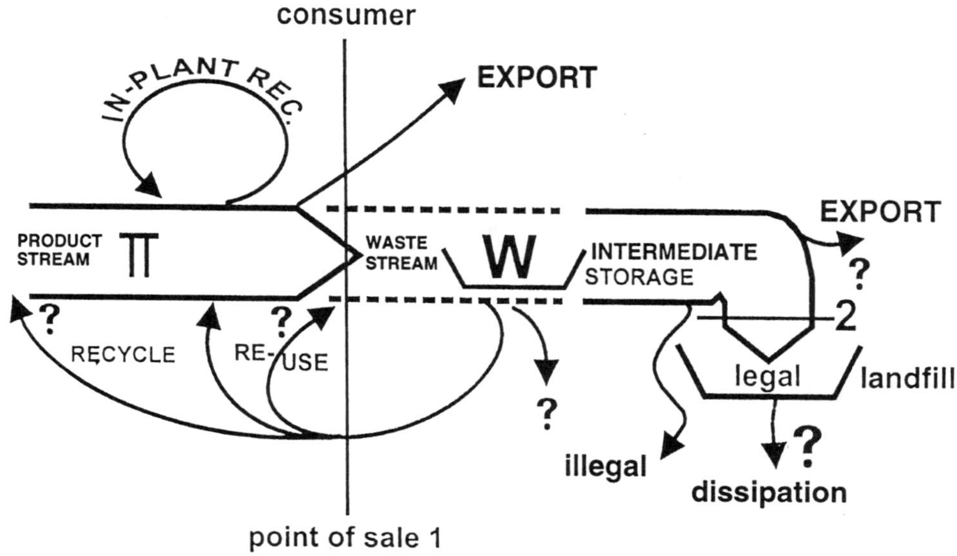


*Figure 6.* Old (pre-1990) waste management: straight-through from production to landfill.

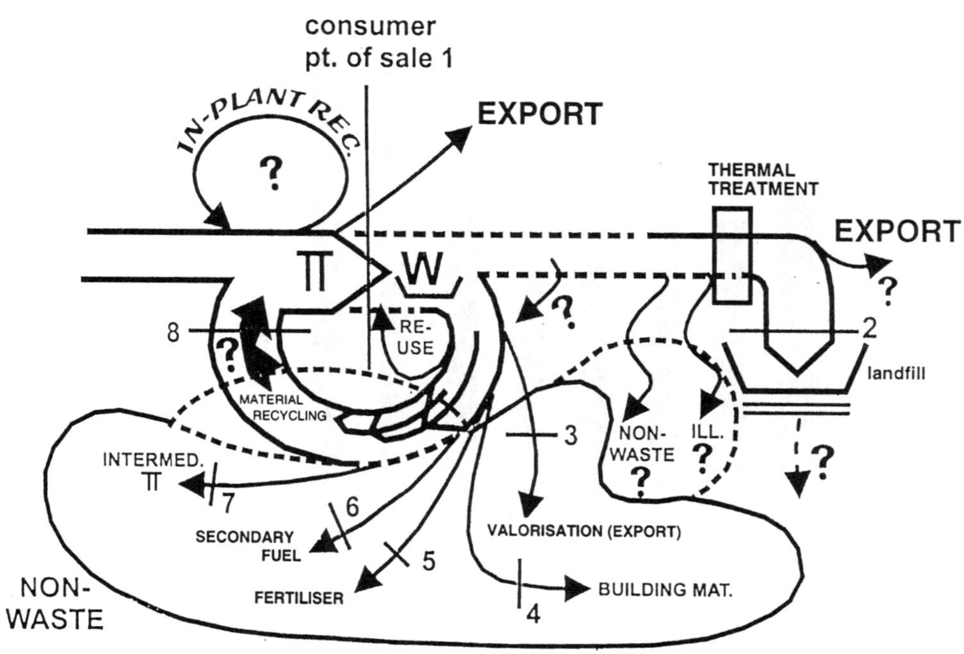


*Figure 7.* New integrated waste management: material recovery, waste/non-waste 'competition'.

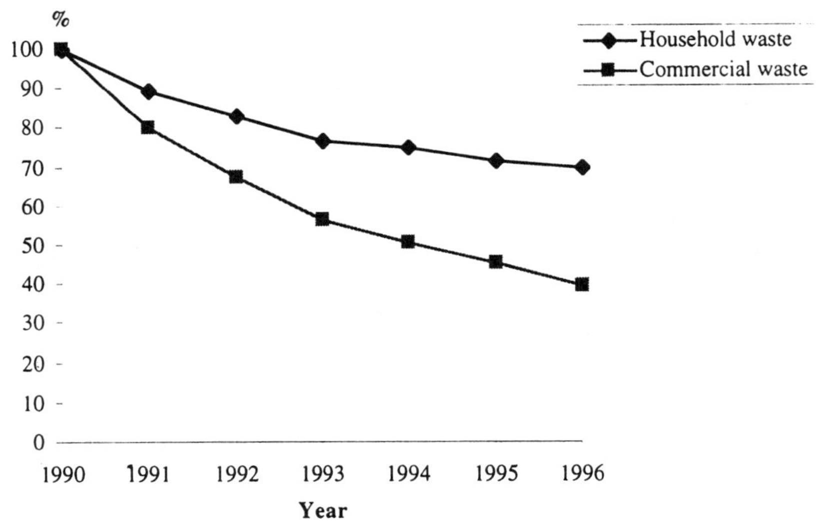


*Figure 8.* The relative vanishing quantities of waste due to recovery options (Steinmetz, Bavaria).

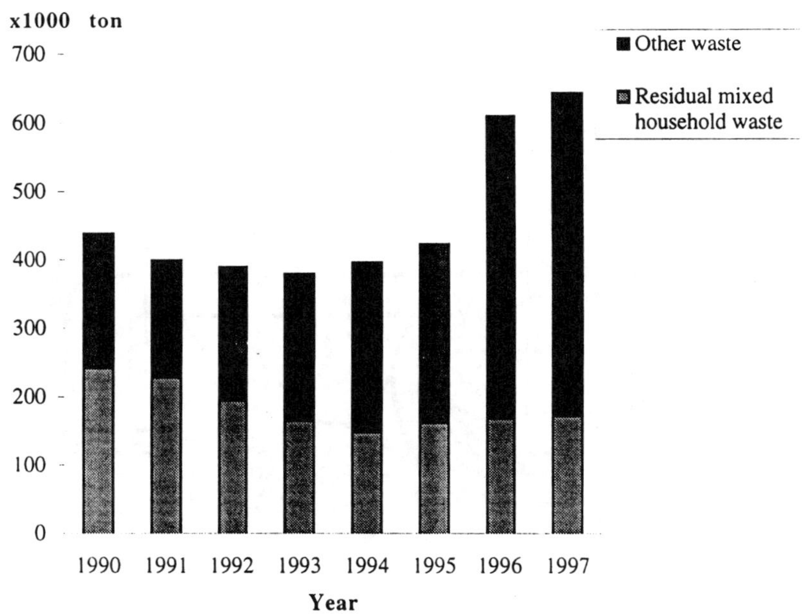


*Figure 9.* Annual waste to Styrian landfills (1990-1997).

According to this philosophy, waste might 'disappear' (cf. Figure 8: decreasing amounts of household wastes and - more drastically - decreasing amounts of commercial waste in

Bavaria/ Germany, where 80 per cent of the combustible waste goes to modern waste incinerators). If no incineration is available, but landfilling is practised ('as far as it goes', in Austria until 2004/2008), residual mixed household waste decreases (cf. Figure 9, Styrian practice). However, the total of mixed household and 'other waste' (presumably separated waste) explains this decrease between 1990 and 1995 (which always used to be about 400,000 to 450,000 tpy in the province of Styria). When others found out about the cheap landfilling practices there was a rush of waste into Styria/Austria amounting to nearly 650,000 tpy!

## 3. Quantifiable Risk Potential of 'Waste'

If 'waste' is incinerated or thermally treated in an up-to-date plant its nature and its composition within the usual variations are unimportant. It is equally unimportant if the 'waste' is labelled 'secondary fuel', 'residual waste', or 'thermal valorisation material' etc. These up-to-date plants are equipped with continuous measurement facilities which document all relevant 'waste incineration parameters', and the technology to observe emissions into the air, effluent water and leachates into the ground. This technology aims at the permanent control of all factors relevant to human health and to the protection of the environment. The complete concept guarantees that the plant acts as a 'sink' for all toxic ingredients in the incinerated products.

Organic toxics are decomposed by combustion; inorganic toxics are concentrated in different compartments (slags, ashes, residues, filter cakes etc., in considerably smaller volumes than in the original input). They can be either recycled or deposited.

## 4. Thermal Treatment of Waste

The environmental and health-relevant aspects of waste incineration were addressed by clean-air acts in different legislations all over Europe (and the EU). This process started in around 1988 and is still on-going. Figure 10 (Löffler, 1984/1988) illustrates the achievement resulting from this legislation and the consequent installation of gas cleaning devices in the three Vienna (Austria) incinerators. The figures show the effect on the reduction of immission of HCl, the most important 'waste gas' which is indicative for the pollution resulting from waste incineration by applying modern gas cleaning.

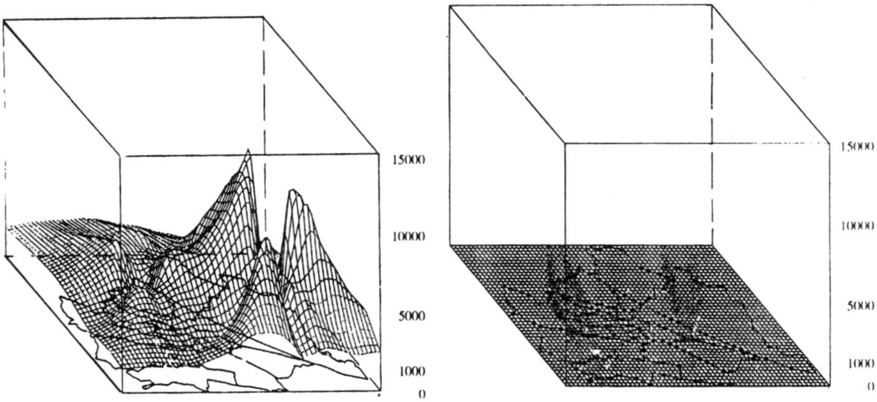


*Figure 10.* HCl-immission situation due to waste incineration in Vienna (MA 22 authority data). Left: situation without modern gas cleaning (winter 1984-85) (ng/m$^3$); right: situation with modern gas cleaning (winter 1987-88) (ng/m$^3$). All other immissions are reduced accordingly to the 'waste incinerator lead gas' HCl.

A modern waste incinerator, which complies with the 0.1 ng TEQ/m$^3$ dioxin-emission standard and good incineration practice, is a sink for organic toxics. A 200,000 tpy waste incinerator decreases the annual 10 g TEQ dioxin content of the waste incinerated to less than 0.05 g of gas emission, less than 0.05 g emission in slag and less than 0.1 g emission through fly ash (Figure 11).[4] Moreover, it has been shown that waste incinerators in member states with a pro-active environmental legislation have not only drastically reduced their dioxin emissions, but they also perform better than many other industrial and private (household!) combustion sources (UNEP, 1999).

An incinerator is also a sink (or collector) for environmentally hazardous heavy metals such as mercury (Hg) and cadmium (Cd). The first is concentrated in the acid washing stage where it is extracted in a concentrated form (filter cake, to be either recycled or deposited underground at a rate of about 1 kg for 1 ton of original waste). Cadmium is concentrated in the filter ash wherefrom it can be extracted by an extra acid wash with the

[4] Editorial footnote: The data presented above and in Figure 11 is a small subset of the total mass balance of a typical incinerator and they should therefore be interpreted with caution. To put this data

same intentions as above for Hg. After waste incineration less than 10 per cent of the original amount of waste needs to be deposited (slags, filter ashes and filter cake, cf. Figure 12).

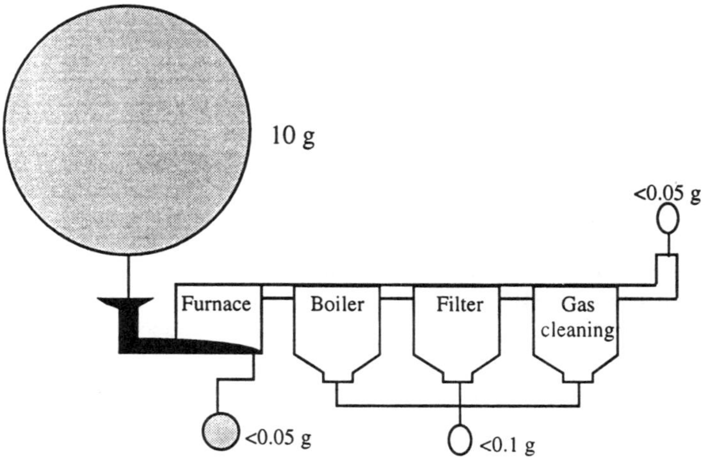


*Figure 11.* The modern waste incinerator as a sink for dioxins (TEQ PCDD/F's in gram per year for a 200,000 tpy municipal waste incinerator) (after Vehlow, 1990).

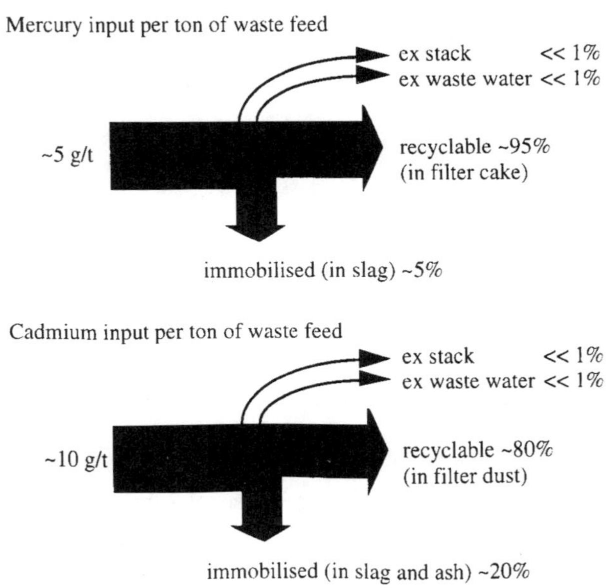


*Figure 12.* The sink for mercury and cadmium in improved waste incinerators.

in full context refer to Figure 23 of Chapter 'Particulate Aerosols, Incinerators and Health').

Equally environmentally relevant is the use of energy resulting from waste incineration. The net energy efficiency (heat and power) contained in waste for an old boiler system, such as the one in Vienna Spittelau, is about 75 per cent (and may be brought up by higher pressure and higher temperature boilers to about 80 per cent).

*Table 11.* Comparison of concentrations/emissions of waste incinerator Spittelau (district heating) to single home heating. (Base: waste incineration 240,000 tpy; 60 $MW_{th}$ + 6 $MW_{el}$ / 80 per cent efficiency).

| | District heating Spittelau | | Single home heating (emission in ton/year) | | | |
|---|---|---|---|---|---|---|
| | Concen-tration °($mg/Nm^3$) *($\mu g/Nm^3$) | Emission (ton/year) | Wood | Coal | Oil | Gas |
| HCl | 9° | 12.96 | No detailed measurements available | | | |
| HF | <0.02° | 0.029 | " | | | |
| $SO_2$ | 14.5° | 20.88 | 44 | 1,560 | 540 | 4 |
| CO | 35° | 50.40 | 30,940 | 23,610 | 380 | 290 |
| $NO_x$ | 86.3° | 124.271 | 110 | 160 | 120 | 130 |
| Org. C | 2.3° | 2.312 | 4,420 | 1,770 | 60 | 40 |
| Dust | 1.4° | 2.016 | 440 | 630 | 20 | 0 |
| Pb | 27.6* | 0.04 | No detailed measurements available | | | |
| Zn | 37.2* | 0.054 | " | | | |
| Cd | 1.5* | 0.0021 | " | | | |
| As | <0.4* | <0.0002 | " | | | |
| Ni | 1.1* | 0.0015 | " | | | |
| Cr | <1.8* | <0.0026 | " | | | |
| Hg | <20* | <0.029 | " | | | |

Waste-to-energy by a co-generation plant (like the one in Vienna Spittelau) results in less air pollution than when the same amount of energy is produced by individual home heating devices (one could truly call this 'less than zero or negative emission'). The comparison provided in Table 11 (Löffler, 1990) shows that, e.g., if waste-to-energy derived district heating was to be substituted for single home heating with wood, emissions for CO would rise from about 50 tpy to 30,940 tpy. Total organic carbon emissions from waste incineration of about 2.3 tpy would increase to 60 tpy when using heating oil in individual home heating. For heavy metals no hard data are available, but considering the single home heating practices in winter one can only guess the positive effect of clean air district heating from waste incineration. For warm countries in southern Europe, district cooling is also a viable option with similar beneficial effects.

Modern incinerator emissions also compare in an interesting way with those of other (incineration/combustion) sources. The incinerator in Wels (Austria) is such a modern plant. It employs higher-order hierarchical waste management features such as a waste recycling park (for collection and material recovery of various goods) and a fly ash treatment unit (allowing the recovery of heavy metals and for the organic treatment of ashes and slags). In total, the new Wels incinerator in Austria compares favourably with emissions from private cars in Wels. Figure 13 shows the comparison between car emissions and waste incinerator emissions. The latter prove to be negligible!

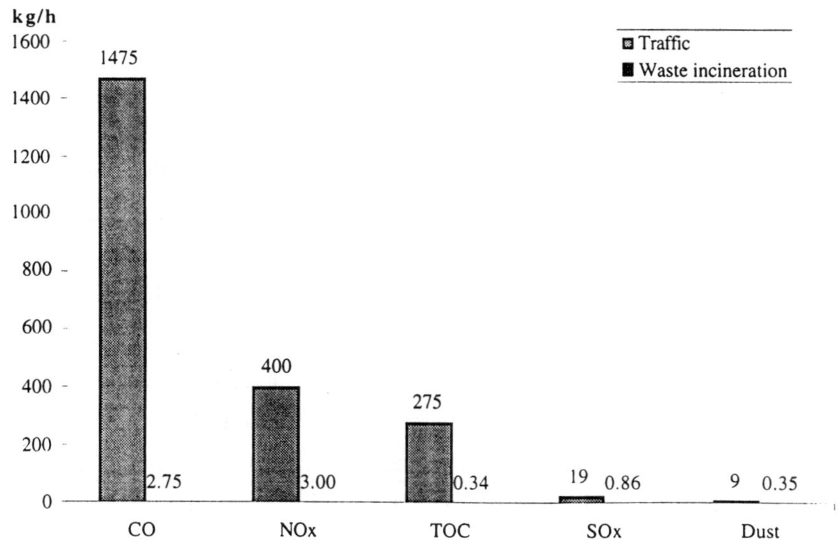


*Figure 13.* Emission comparison between city traffic (5000 cars) and the municipal waste incinerator in Wels, Austria (hourly emission in kg).

The administration and competent authorities in Austria also acted on 'public acceptance'. Two examples of this concern (a) a project by Hundertwasser, a world-famous 'green' architect, who made the outside of the Spittelau incinerator in Vienna an international renowned 'showcase' (after having been convinced himself that this modern waste incinerator was the best ecological solution), and (b) on-line emission data of the relevant pollutants emitted are on public display at the Spittelau gate.

Costs of incineration are commonly exaggerated by referencing to bad examples (which indeed exist). They often have to do with poor planning, over-dimensioning of incinerators, or insecure politicians changing the exploitation plan in an unforeseen way. Waste incinerator costs concern mainly the financing of the plant (investment-cost) ; only about 20 to 25 per cent are operational costs. The financial issue is often clouded by considering 'tariffs' and 'taxes' as 'costs' (public utilities). In Bavaria (Germany) 80 per cent of household waste is incinerated in technically high standard waste incinerators. The average cost per family is 400 DM per year, or roughly 1 DM per family per day; the costs per ton increase to DM 800/t of waste treated. In many cases the higher figures relate to places *without* a waste incinerator! Moreover, the costs for incineration should be related to those of the contaminated land restoration and cleaning-up of leaking landfills.

## 5. Guidelines to Solve the 'Waste Problem'

1. Combustible waste has important potential energy. On the other hand it contains harmful and toxic substances. In Austria, the 'ASTRA' - The Impact of Selected Scenarios of Thermal Waste Treatment on the Environment in Austria - report has investigated which processes provide optimal utilisation of combustible waste for waste-to-energy within the frame of the Austrian waste management law - AWG (Brunner *et al.*, 1998). For this evaluation the principle of material flow analysis was used. This approach allows the determination of 'transfer factors' for (toxic) materials in various thermal treatment processes (mono- and co-incineration plants). Questions addressed include: into which matrix will a toxic substance (e.g. cadmium) be transferred and can this matrix be considered as ecologically sound, i.e. is this a sink, concentrating this toxic material or is it a diffuse path that is followed?

   This study has shown the need for more specific investigations on different aspects of co-incineration, especially in the cement industry, for which there is an ensuing study (PRIZMA, Brunner 1999, shortly to be published); other sectoral studies, e.g. for wood residues, may follow.

The ASTRA-study concluded that using all 8.5 million tons of Austrian combustible waste per year, the emissions to the atmosphere will decrease by 43 per cent over today's practice, despite the fact that 2.3 times more waste will be incinerated in this scenario than today.

2. Waste is an heterogeneous material. Therefore, defining sampling and analysing is difficult. Moreover, there is an important financial interest to substitute waste by 'non-waste'-material or other labels seeking cheaper waste handling and treatment routes. For all these reasons, there should be more than an 'annual', one-time check on all sorts of emissions to enforce compliance for users of non-standard/secondary fuels, but a continuous measurement of the main parameters with alike standards for dedicated waste incinerators and industrial co-incineration.

   A practical possibility for enforcing this compliance, especially for co-incineration plants, is envisaged by 'continuous gas-monitoring' whereby key waste gas indicators such as HCl are measured on a continuous monitoring basis. The continuous sampling of dioxins, with a measurement relating to two or three weeks of sampling is also possible in this context.

3. A permanent European discussion platform of experts debating on practical rules and waste treatment guidelines, might be advantageous. Such a body should be complementary to the actual legislatory guidelines, both the ones which are accepted and the ones under discussion (Waste Incineration Directive/ common position 9635/99 of June 30, 1999). Participants could be members of various institutions, such as the European Commission, the involved industrial sectors, government authorities, environmental NGO's, and consumer groups. The scope of the work could cover among others: waste qualities, substances in waste, plant-related materials, 'positive lists', monitoring-practices, credentials, health findings etc. The aim should be more coherence on these issues in the member states. ASPIS may prove to be a useful platform for this type of information exchange.

4. The increased efforts by the EU-parliament (e.g., Doc. A4-223/(98) to set up 'sustainable economies' (also for 'waste management') are worth mentioning. Sustainable economical management of waste can only have an impact on environmental quality when clear and practical rules are enforced in a visible way. Moreover, standards should be similar for all players and complied with in line with continuous checks, of which the results are advertised in an accessible way.

## Acknowledgement

The newly formed European Committee of the national trade organisations of the Environmental Technology Suppliers Associations EUCETSA, of which I act as vice-chairman and head of the waste management working group, will clearly follow up in promoting awareness of the environmental benefits of environmental technologies. We welcome any practical considerations dealing with the enforcement of practical and controllable rules to truly implement environmental technology as a source of active protection of the environment.

We are most grateful for the discussion started by ASPIS. This platform aims at contributing to continuous improvement on the road to knowledge and awareness on environmental health. This is a proper and relevant area for waste treatment discussion.

## References

Bontoux and Leone (1997) Waste management IPTS report EUR 17716-EN, Seville, Spain, November 1997.

Brunner, P.H., Fehringer, R., Rechberger, H., and Personen, H. (1998) *ASTRA Study*, IWAS Institute, Technical University of Vienna.

De Fodor, E. (1911) *Elektrizität aus Kehricht*, K.U.K. Hofbuchhandlung von Julius Benkö, Budapest.

EU (1996) Community Strategy for waste management, COM (96) 399 EU.

EU Waste Framework Directive 75/442/EEC as amended by 91/156/EEC.

Jägerhuber, G. (1997, 1998) Report Styrian Government's waste management report.

Kneissl, P. (1990) WAV, Comparison of emissions of Wels city traffic with MSWI emissions, permitting data.

Löffler, H. (1984/1988) HCl immission analysis by Vienna Magistrate Air Pollution Protection Dept., MA22, Vienna, Austria.

Löffler, H. (1990) *Comparison of Concentrations/Emissions MSWI Spittelau with Single Home Heating (Wood, Coal, Heating Oil, Gas)*, UTEC, Vienna, Austria.

Steinmetz, H.C. (1998) Vanishing waste quantities in *Thermische Abfall-behandlung*, Garching.

United Nations Environment Programme – UNEP (1999) *Dioxin and Furan Inventories*, Geneva, Switzerland.

Vehlow, J. (1990) *PCDD/F Destruction in a Modern Waste Incinerator*, JRC Forschungszentrum, Karlsruhe, Germany.

# POLICY OPTIONS FOR WASTE MANAGEMENT IN GREECE

*The Hellenic National Solid Waste Management Plan*

C. DONTAS
*Ministry of Environmental Housing Planning and Public Works*
*Parnasidos 57*
*Chalandri*
*15321 Athens*
*GREECE*

**Summary**

Until recently, waste management in Greece was non-existent. This paper is an overview of the fundamental changes in waste management policy the country must undertake.

The first part analyses the basic data on which a waste management policy should be built. It highlights the urban-rural-mountainous areas-islands dimension of the problem, the amount of waste which is produced and the relevant policy trends from abroad.

Household waste management options are: recycling and composting, and up-to-date, well-equipped sanitary landfills of which minimal use will be made. The policy also involves the sanitation of existing black-spots, which are the result of contamination from waste deposit sites which were inappropriately localised and badly managed in the past. Greece has not decided to take the incineration option and might put more stress on prevention in the future.



*P. Nicolopoulou-Stamati et al. (eds.), Health Impacts of Waste Management Policies*, 107–120.

75 per cent of hospital waste is managed by two specialised centres in Athens and Thessaloniki. As regards the remaining 25 per cent, cost-effective options need to be established which take the dispersion of the problem into account.

The Greek authorities deal with industrial waste in the same way as they handle household waste: reduction of quantities and especially of harmful substances, recycling and safe handling. As eighty per cent of the problem is localised in only twenty industrial organisations, agreements on waste management along these lines were established with these companies.

However, this innovative waste management plan, which is in line with the EU Directives and with the policies in other member countries, needs substantial funding, of which only one quarter has been approved. There is serious doubt as to the provenance and the availability of the remaining three-quarters.

## 1. Introduction

During the past few years the issue of waste management has undergone a mild change. Consumption patterns have developed in a way which creates more waste. In addition to the increasing amounts of waste, there has also been a change in quality, e.g. due to increasing amounts of plastics, waste has become less and less degradable. To deal with this development, considerable experience, technology and funding is needed (Markatos *et al.*, 1998; Galetas, 1991).

In the past, Greece never faced serious environmental problems concerning waste. However, this has changed during the past decade with increased tourism, and also with changing consumption patterns in Greek society. Greece is now forced to come up with solutions which take into account the peculiarities that appear in the country.

This paper reviews the policy waste management intentions in Greece. It starts by analysing the basic data for this policy. Different approaches exist for household, hospital and industrial waste. The last part of the paper looks into the financing of this innovative policy, which is in line with the EU options[5].

## 2. Dimensions of the Waste Problem in Greece

Greece has 10 million inhabitants. The Greater Athens area (Attica) holds 40 per cent of the population of the country, 45 per cent of industry and 60 per cent of the social services. These are concentrated in an area that is roughly 4 per cent of the total size of the country (Regional Association of Municipalities and Communities of Attica, 1993). A similar concentration of activities is found in the other two major urban centres, Thessaloniki and Patras. Consequently, a specific waste policy design is needed to take the major urban centres into account (Figure 14).

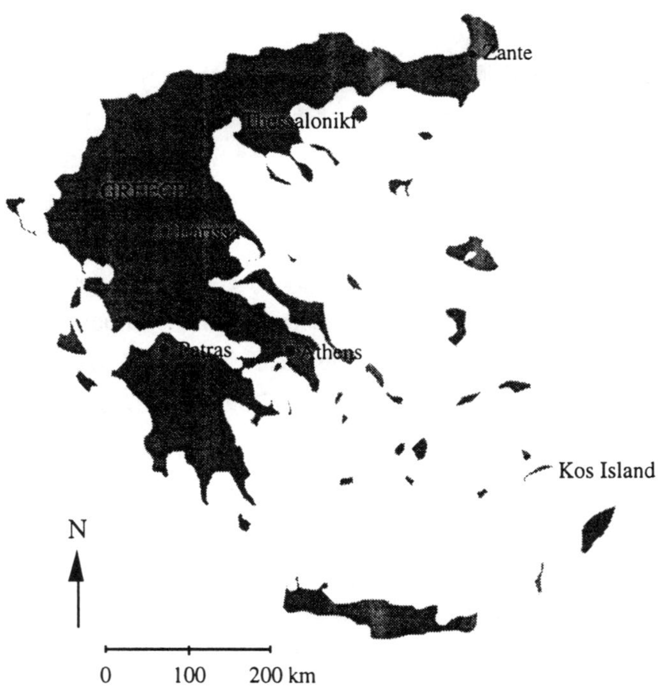


*Figure 14.* Map of Greece.

---

[5] Dir. 74/442, OJ 15/07/1975; Dir. 91/156, OJ 18/03/1991; Dir. 78/319, OJ 20/03/1978; Dir. 91/689.

Secondly, Greece has three thousand five hundred islands which, during the summertime, are visited by a lot of tourists and consequently, significant amounts of waste are generated as compared to wintertime. Waste policy in Greece needs to deal with this seasonal increase of waste.

A third and fourth area of concern are the rural areas and the mountainous regions of the country.

In conclusion, from a waste policy point of view, Greece consists of four different geomorphologic areas, each with its own specific needs.

In setting up a waste management plan one further needs to consider:

- the current situation;
- the available technology;
- the financial resources, subject to financial management and conscious choices;
- the acclimatisation and familiarisation of the public with waste programmes to promote acceptance. The participation of the public in a new policy is crucial for its success. (Experience world-wide has shown that it is of key importance to involve the general public at the earliest possible time.)

This paper describes in general terms the programme which the Greek Ministry for the Environment intends to implement. It serves as an example of a policy for a specific, up-to-date and so-called alternative waste management system. The data are gathered in the Hellenic National Solid Waste Management Plan (Dontas and Loizidou, 1998).

Until 1994 waste management in Greece was in its preliminary phase. At that time, the country had a total of three and a half thousand authorised waste disposal sites. Research on one thousand, four hundred and twenty of these sites showed that 50 per cent of them were found to be located in areas where the soil is permeable for the leachate. Therefore these sites are unsuitable. Of the remainder, 19 per cent were located in areas where the soil is semi-permeable. Only 31 per cent of the landfills were located in geologically suitable areas.

Today, Greece produces yearly 3.1 million tons of household waste, 450,000 tons of industrial waste and roughly 15,000 tons of hospital waste. Both this quantity and the sites where they are dumped constitute a huge problem that has to be managed. One of the keys is the composition of the waste, which for household waste is shown in Table 12.

*Table 12.* Household waste composition (in %) in Greece (1990).

| **Fraction** | % |
|---|---|
| Organic material | 47 |
| Paper | 20 |
| Plastic | 9 |
| Metal | 4.5 |
| Glass | 4.5 |
| Remaining fraction | 15 |

Figure 15 provides more details on these data and points to the evolution during the period 1984-1990 (Papachristou, 1998; Regional Association of Communities and Municipalities of Attica, 1990). The data indicate that almost half is organic material which can be composted. Note, however, the relative amount decreased from almost 60 per cent in 1984 to 48 per cent 1990. Paper makes up 20 per cent of the total weight. Although plastic represented only 10 per cent of the total weight in 1990, its relative contribution doubled over a six-year period.

At this point, a comparison with the national programme for waste management up to the year 2000 in the USA and the EU policy lines might be useful. In the US, during the period 1980-2000, the quantity of waste to be landfilled will remain constant. Increasing amounts will be recycled. Most remarkably the programme also foresees that the amount to be incinerated has increased 7 times during the last 20 years (Figure 16) (Dontas, 1999).

The data for the year 1990 in Europe show that 60 per cent of waste is deposited in sanitary landfills. Of the remaining part, 16 per cent is incinerated and the remaining 24 per cent has to be recycled.

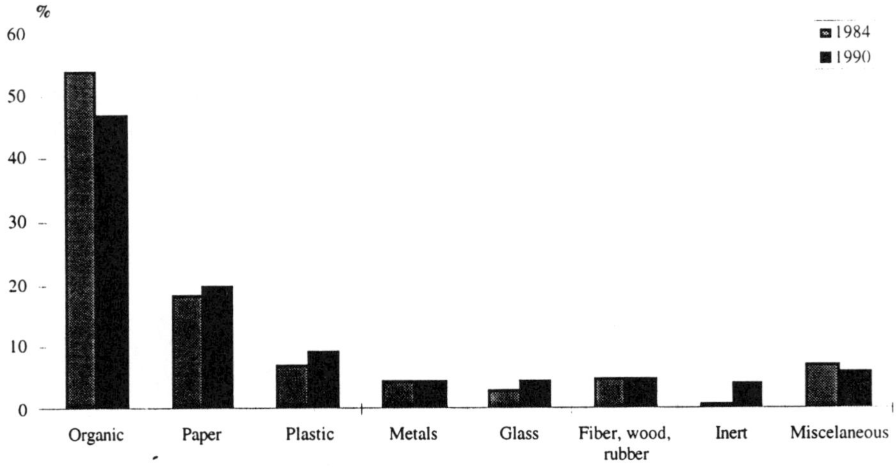


*Figure 15.* Composition of solid household waste in Greece (weight %). Comparison is made between the 1984 and the 1990 data.

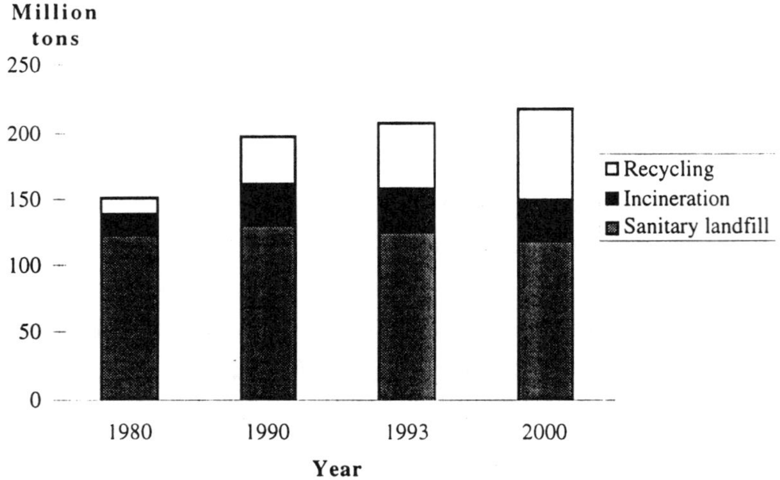


*Figure 16.* Evolution of the management options for municipal solid waste in the USA during the period 1980-1993. Forecast for the year 2000.

Table 13 provides waste treatment data for selected industrialised countries. Although Austria recycles 24 per cent of its waste, the table shows that the country still manages 60 per cent of its household waste through sanitary landfill.

*Table 13.* Percentage of household waste quantities landfilled, incinerated and recycled in different countries (data for the period 1988-1990).

| Country | Sanitary landfills (%) | Incineration (%) | Recycling (%) |
|---|---|---|---|
| EU | 60 | 33 | 7 |
| Switzerland | 18 | 80 | 2 |
| Norway | 65 | 23 | 12 |
| Sweden | 35 | 60 | 5 |
| Japan | 24 | 74 | 2 |
| USA | 75 | 15 | 10 |
| Austria | 60 | 16 | 24 |
| Poland | 99 | - | 1 |
| Hungary | 88 | 11 | 1 |
| Canada | 96 | 4 | - |

Switzerland, Sweden and Japan incinerate more than half of their household waste. In most countries, however, incineration accounts for less than one third of the waste treatment. The most prevalent option is still landfilling, with 60 per cent (W/W) in the EU, and 96 per cent (W/W) in Canada. Candidate EU countries such as Poland and Hungary deposit 88 to 99 per cent of their waste in (uncontrolled) landfills.

## 3. Household Waste Policy Options

In Greece, recycling is an important issue, as is conservation of energy from the production of recycled items. In this context, the energy 'recycled' from incinerators is debatable from an efficiency point of view. The energy needed to reproduce the incinerated item is four times higher than the energy which is generated from its incineration. For example, to produce 1 kg of paper one needs an amount of energy which is four times higher than the energy provided during the incineration of this 1 kg of paper. Moreover, incineration also entails the pollution of the atmosphere and the production of highly contaminated liquids and ashes. Greece, just like other countries, faces a problem finding suitable areas for sanitary landfills. Incineration contributes to this problem, as 15 to 20 per cent of the original material turns into ash which needs to be landfilled in (the rare) suitable deposit sites (Galetas, 1991).

The second option concerns the production of compost (Christoulas and Kapetanios, 1989; Kapetanios and Drougas, 1992; Kapetanios *et al.*, 1999). Greek waste is 47 per cent organic material. Composting is possible as the available technology is up-to-date, both for aerobic and anaerobic decomposition and simultaneous production of energy. The odour problem, inevitably linked to composting, can be managed. Compost of good quality necessitates sufficient phosphorous and nitrogen at a proper rate. This aspect can be controlled. Also sludge will be composted. Following these two operations, it is assumed that 25 per cent will be left over, which can be deposited in a safe way in sanitary landfills.

The sanitary landfill in Patras has a clay protection layer 50 cm thick. On top of that, a membrane has been placed, and, on top of the membrane, there is a cloth which is, in turn, covered with clay once more. This system provides full soil protection and the area has an opening to collect rainwater and avoid flooding. The water percolating through the site is collected by a drainage system and biologically treated (Loizidou *et al.*, 1992; Loizidou and Kapetanios, 1993). After a few years the waste produces a considerable amount of biogas (Kapetanios and Loizidou, 1996). The system allows the collection of this gas, which, in turn, is used to generate electricity. In the first few years, however, gas production is too limited for recycling. This system has not only been installed in Patras, but also in Thessaloniki, Zante and Larissa. It serves as a model for the rest of the country.

In co-ordination with local authorities, a few areas in Greece were selected and sanitary landfills have been set up or are about to be realised. One cannot start a recycling programme and ignore the residue that results from it; rather, one is forced to classify the materials and start from the basic structure. In the years to come (2000-2005), rigorous recycling programmes will take off in Greece. Such programmes will include either mechanical collection and sorting in appropriate plants, or inexpensive, selective collection at source (Sypsas, 1995; Skordilis, 1991). Production centres for compost will be built in every region of Greece.

## 4. Policy Options for Industrial and Hospital Waste (Kapetanios, 1990)

In addition to household waste, there are significant amounts of both industrial and hospital waste.

Currently, there are twenty-nine thousand hospital beds in Athens, seven thousand eight hundred and sixty in Thessaloniki and the remaining twenty thousand are found in the other parts of the country (Figure 17). All together they produce 15,000 tons of hospital waste a year. Research has shown that dealing with the hospital waste of Athens and Thessaloniki is 75 per cent of the problem (Kapetanios, 1999).

Two centres of hospital waste management have been approved: one in Attica and the other in Thessaloniki. They deal with three quarters of the hospital waste of the country. For the remaining 25 per cent, such as that of the isle of Kos, which is in a remote area, safe ways of managing waste need to be found, ways in which hospital waste is dealt with on the same basis as household waste. A crucial issue here is sterilisation. This can be done either by radiation or by steam treatment, but specific European guidelines are lacking. This causes inertia in choosing between these technologies.

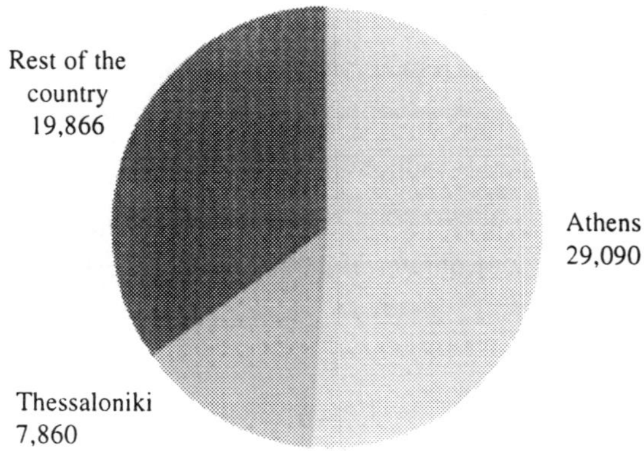


*Figure 17.* Distribution of hospital beds in Greece (1998) (Number of beds).

Greece also produces 450,000 tons of industrial waste annually (Dontas *et al.*, 1998). This amount does not necessitate large treatment plants. The problem originates from twenty major factories producing 80 per cent of the industrial waste. The Ministry for the Environment reached an agreement with these factories. It means that they will adopt strategies aiming at:

- the reduction of the use of substances that might be dangerous through technological changes;
- the reduction of the volume of the produced waste by adopting clean technologies;
- the recycling of the materials which are produced and an increase in their life-cycle;
- safe handling of the remaining waste through specific technologies. An example of this are dialytes not containing chloride. This material can be used by the cement industry, in which case it does not cause major atmospheric emissions.

## 5. Financial Concerns

These programmes have an economic cost which is currently largely unknown. Moreover, it is unknown who will pay for it. 4.2 billion Drachmas (US$ 13.4 million - 12.8 MEuro) has been approved for Attica (the capital region), 21 billion Drachmas (US$ 67.2 million – 63.9 MEuro) for Thessaloniki and 35 billion Drachmas (US$ 112.0 million – 106.5 MEuro) for the remaining parts of the country (Figure 18). At this moment the total amount of money provided for waste policy in Greece does not exceed 100 billion Drachmas (US$ 320.0 million - 304.2 MEuro). This sum is provided by the Greek authorities and the EU collaboration via multiple funding. More money is required, since the amount covers only one quarter of the projected necessary funding for the period 2000-2005.

According to the Greek Ministry of the Environment, an adequate solution to the waste problems in the country by the year 2005 necessitates an investment plan of up to 380 billion Drachmas (US$ 1,216.1 million – 1,156.1 MEuro), which needs to be spent during the next five years.

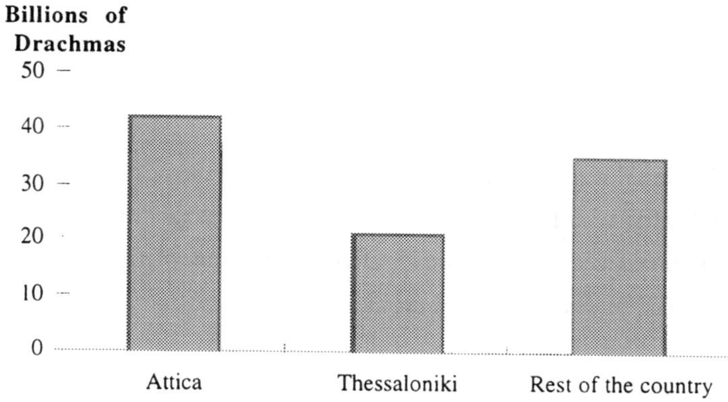


*Figure 18.* Financial resources spend to the waste management policy in Greece during the period 1994-1999.

The first phase of the plan entails setting up sanitary landfills to stop the leakage of water into rivers, lakes and the groundwater resources.

Another sum of money has been allocated to deal with the decontamination of historic black-spots. This has an important social aspect as it addresses those areas which have suffered serious damage in the past. It is indeed the responsibility of both the state and the citizenry to restore them and to give them back to the general public. For this reason a huge programme has been developed in the region of Attica, where for twenty-five years 2,500 acres of polluted soil have been absorbing the waste of Athens and the surrounding area.

The third phase deals with installing the infrastructure for the recycling systems and compost production. This will also fulfil Greece's responsibilities to the existing EU Directives.

## 6. Conclusions

Household waste policy in Greece aims at limiting waste disposal and repairing the environmental damage done by inappropriate waste disposal in the past. Central to the new approach is recycling with special emphasis on composting. In this way over 50 per cent of the current household waste stream can be managed. Incineration is not an option. New deposit sites will be established and managed according to the most advanced technologies.

75 per cent of hospital waste problems are concentrated in the large urban areas of Athens and Thessaloniki. In each of these areas a thermal treatment facility has been organised to treat the contaminated water. Small scale, effective and inexpensive treatment, especially on the islands, constitutes an unsolved problem.

Industrial waste is minimised through agreements with the main plants, which produce 80 per cent of the waste in the country.

Waste management in Greece therefore does not differ substantially from the mainstream options in other EU countries. It arrived later than in other EU countries, but is characterised by specific issues as regards incineration. Also the prevention option needs to be further established.

At the end of a five year investment plan, by the year 2005 Greece will have up-to-date waste management which will safeguard the environment in a considerably more efficient way.

## References

Christoulas, K., and Kapetanios, E.G. (1989) Composting management in Attica Region, Regional Association of Communities and Municipalities of Attica, Greece, Internal Report.

Dontas, K.N. (1999) Proceedings in regulation and legislation in Greece, Seventh International Waste Management and Landfill Symposium, University of Cagliary, Italy.

Dontas, K.N., and Loizidou, M.D. (1998) *Hellenic National Solid Waste Management Planning*, Ministry of Environment, Housing Planning and Public Works, Athens, Greece.

Galetas, N. (1991) Technical and economical comparison of waste management methods, Internal Report, Ministry of Internal Affairs, Greece.

Kapetanios, E.G. (1990) Methods and techniques for hazardous waste treatment and disposal, in *Proceedings on the Conference for Industrial Activities and Environment*, Hellenic Chemical Engineering Union, pp. 193-205.

Kapetanios, E.G. (1999) Construction of incineration plant for the hospital waste in Attica, Regional Association of Communities and Municipalities of Attica, Greece, Internal Report.

Kapetanios, E.G., and Drougas, A.D. (1992) The problem of sewage sludge and management of Psittalia's island wastewater treatment plant in Attica, *Acta Horticulture* **301**, 105-111.

Kapetanios, E.G., and Loizidou, M.D. (1996) Evaluation of the landfill site as a reserve source for biogas production, Regional Association of Communities and Municipalities of Attica and University of Athens, Greece, Internal Report.

Kapetanios, E.G., Katsoulis, A.A., and Gavathas, A.D. (1999) Cost-benefit analysis for the mechanical recycling and composting plant in Attica, Regional Association of Communities and Municipalities of Attica, Greece, Internal Report.

Loizidou, M.D., Vilthoulkas, N., and Kapetanios, E.G. (1992) Physical-chemical treatment of leachate from landfills, *J. Environmental Science and Health* **27** (**4**), 245-250.

Loizidou, M.D., and Kapetanios, E.G. (1993) Effect of leachate from landfills on underground water quality, *The Science of the Total Environment* **128**, 69-81.

Markatos, N., Loizidou, M.D., and Kapetanios, E.G. (1998) Comparative evaluation of different technologies for waste management, Internal Report, National Technical University of Athens, Greece.

Papachristou, E. (1998) Analysis of household waste in the greater area of Thessaloniki, Internal Report, Department of Chemical Engineering, Aristotelian University of Thessaloniki, Greece.

Regional Association of Communities and Municipalities of Attica (1990) Analysis of household waste in the Greater Area of Athens, Greece, Internal Report.

Regional Association of Communities and Municipalities of Attica (1993) Regional solid waste management in Attica, Greece, Internal Report.

Skordilis, A. (1991) Recycling of paper, glass and aluminium in Greece, Ministry of Environment, Housing Planning and Public Works, Internal Report.

Sypsas, K. (1995) *Recycling in Greece*, International Organisation of Biopolitics.

# WASTE MANAGEMENT POLICIES IN THE UNITED STATES OF AMERICA

G. VALAORAS
*University of La Verne*
*Athens Campus*
*PO Box 51105*
*14510 Kifissia*
*GREECE*

## Summary

Waste management has become a major environmental management problem in recent years, as the quantity of waste streams increases and grows in complexity: the result of an ever-widening range of products in our consumer-based society. Hazardous waste in particular has been subject to detailed and costly regulations since the early 1980's, when unregulated toxic wastes were associated with profound health effects in exposed populations at Love Canal, New York and Times Beach, Missouri. The legislative response in the United States has been comprehensive, yet a whole list of problems still exist which need more sophisticated management within the US regulatory framework. The United States regulates waste in terms of two broad categories, hazardous waste and municipal solid waste. The two categories together generated about 422 million tons during the year 1995-96. Solid waste is not considered hazardous, despite the fact that it contains household hazardous waste. Although household waste is, in fact, a mixture of inert and toxic components, it is regulated as municipal solid waste, without the strict federal regulations which apply to hazardous waste.



*P. Nicolopoulou-Stamati et al. (eds.), Health Impacts of Waste Management Policies*, 121–131.

Through the US Environmental Protection Agency (EPA), the federal government implements laws which deal with releases of hazardous substances that may endanger public health, welfare, or the environment. To evaluate the magnitude and hazard of such releases, the EPA has developed risk assessment procedures. Quantitative risk assessment is a methodology used to evaluate hazards, exposures, and the probability of health effects on target populations.

This brief review of waste management policies in the United States describes some of the current issues in risk-based decision-making, and of risk assessment methodology developed at the EPA over the past twenty-five years. Risk assessment methodology is still evolving and is constantly being refined as scientific evidence becomes available. It recently has been expanded to deal with ecological risk, and is used to quantify risks to a wide range of health effects in humans as well as in plants and animals. Most environmental regulations in the US dealing with toxic releases are based on this methodology.

## 1. Waste Management in the United States

The United States regulates wastes in terms of two broad categories, hazardous waste and municipal solid wastes. The two categories together generated about 422 million tons during the year 1995-96, divided approximately equally. The rate of waste generation is more than double the average per capita waste production in Europe. Hazardous waste consists of 97 per cent wastewater, and therefore the major part of it, comprising 143 million tons, is treated in wastewater treatment plants. Another 24 million tons is removed by deep well underground injection, 4 million tons are combusted[6] and one million tons are landfilled. The remaining 42 million tons of hazardous waste are subjected to partial treatment (US EPA, 1998) (Figure 19).

Of 208 million tons of municipal solid waste generated in the year 1995-1996, 119 million tons were landfilled, 56 million tons were recycled, and 34 million tons were

[6] In this chapter preference has been given to the term 'combustion' over the term 'incineration'.

combusted in high temperature incinerators (US EPA, 1998) (Figure 20). Solid waste is not considered hazardous, despite the fact that it contains household hazardous waste.

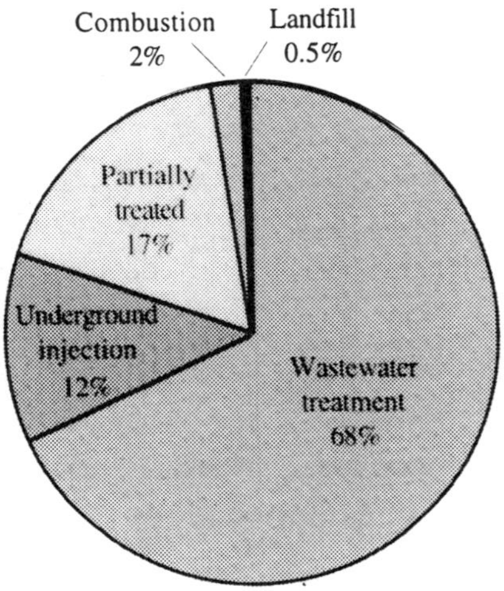


*Figure 19.* Hazardous waste treatment in the US (1995-1996) (after US EPA, 1998).

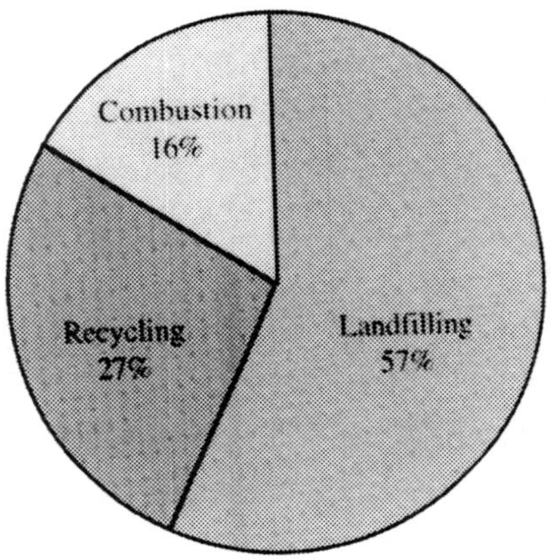


*Figure 20.* Municipal solid waste treatment in the US (1995-1996) (after US EPA, 1998).

Products in the home which are considered hazardous include the following:

- Drain cleaners
- Oven cleaners
- Wood and metal cleaners and polishers
- Automotive oil and fuel additives
- Grease and rust solvents
- Carburettor and fuel injection cleaners
- Air conditioning refrigerants
- Starter fluids
- Paint thinners
- Paint strippers and removers
- Adhesives
- Herbicides
- Pesticides
- Fungicides and wood preservatives (US EPA, 1986)

The only possibilities for removing household hazardous waste from the waste stream are voluntary programmes instituted at state, county or city level. Collection programmes for hazardous household waste are operated at local and state level. Recycling programmes are also voluntary from the point of view of the federal government, and are implemented by states or smaller communities.

A recent review of the health effects associated with populations living near municipal landfill sites gives support to the need to manage hazardous household waste separately from ordinary municipal waste (REHW, 1998). Diseases such as bladder cancer, leukaemia, and lung cancer appear elevated in such populations compared to controls in a variety of geographical locations. Increases in birth defects have also been reported. According to Peter Montague, the editor of Rachel's Environment and Health Weekly, landfill gas consists of naturally occurring methane and carbon dioxide, which are formed when waste decomposes. As pressure builds up inside the landfill, the gases are forced upwards and carry with them toxic chemicals such as paint thinners, solvents, pesticides and other polychlorinated volatile organic compounds.

Montague states in his review:

> *'It should come as no surprise that living near a landfill is hazardous to your health – and it doesn't matter whether the landfill holds solid waste or hazardous waste. Hazardous waste landfills hold unwanted toxic residues from manufacturing processes. On the other hand, municipal solid waste landfills hold discarded products, many of which were manufactured from toxic materials. The wastes go out the back door of the factory while the products go out the front door, but after they have been buried in the ground both wastes and products create very similar hazards for the environment, wildlife, and humans. The leachate (liquid) produced inside the two kinds of landfills is chemically identical.'*
>
> (REHW, 1998)

## 2. Risk Assessment Methodology

Several laws have been instituted which authorise the federal government to deal with releases or threatened releases of hazardous substances that may endanger public health, welfare or the environment. To evaluate cost-effective and scientifically-based responses to the release of hazardous substances, the US Environmental Protection Agency has developed risk assessment procedures. Risk assessment has developed over the last twenty-five years in the field of environmental health sciences, in order to quantify the risks of exposure to toxic or radioactive substances. At the US Environmental Protection Agency (EPA), risk assessments are widely used to contribute to regulatory decisions, and have become a sophisticated tool to prioritise decisions affecting chemicals or chemical products. When such substances are used in commerce, their control or restriction, as well as their eventual disposal, have serious economic consequences. Thus risk assessments are applied in order to provide a consistent evaluation of public health risk.

According to EPA's Guidelines for Carcinogen Risk Assessment, risk assessment defines the adverse health consequences of exposure to toxic agents (EPA, 1987).

Risk assessment includes one or more of the following components: hazard identification, dose-response assessment, exposure assessment and risk characterisation (NRC, 1983). The results of the risk assessment are then integrated with economic, social and political considerations to develop risk management options.

*Hazard identification* is the process of determining whether exposure to the toxic agent has the potential to cause adverse health effects. In the case of a carcinogenic response, the hazard identification includes both malignant and benign tumours manifested in standard toxicological tests such as long-term animal bioassays. A review of physical-chemical properties and routes of exposure, structure-activity relationships, pharmacokinetic properties, and short-term tests, are also elements of the hazard identification. Where clinical or epidemiological studies exist, these increase the weight of evidence for the carcinogenic potential of a toxic agent. Specialised toxicity studies on teratology or mutagenicity also contribute to the determination of adverse health effects.

The *dose-response assessment* is a quantitative assessment of the relationship between the dose and response in the region of human exposure. Carcinogenic compounds are assumed to have no threshold where the risk of cancer is zero. Thus, in the case of cancer incidence, the dose-response assessment uses mathematical extrapolation to estimate risks at low levels of exposure, which cannot be measured directly by animal experiments or epidemiological studies. EPA uses a linearised multistage procedure, which leads to a plausible upper limit to risks. Such an estimate does not necessarily give a realistic prediction of the risks, but gives an upper limit which is unlikely to be exceeded. The potential for carcinogenicity is measured by a cancer potency factor, estimated from toxicity tests.

For non-cancer effects, the EPA assumes there is a threshold for exposure to cause adverse health effects, such as organ damage or reproductive effects. It is assumed that a no adverse effect level (NOAEL) exists, and based on this, a reference dose, or RfD, is determined for each chemical substance. The reference dose is an estimate with an uncertainty of one order of magnitude or more, of a lifetime dose which is likely to be without significant risk to human populations. RfD's and carcinogenic potency factors are developed at EPA for specific chemicals, after extensive peer review.

*Exposure assessment* estimates the exposures to which the population is subject. It includes estimates of the magnitude, duration and frequency of exposure, as well as the potential for exposure via inhalation, ingestion, and dermal penetration. Calculations of absorption through each of these routes assist in quantifying the total exposure from hazardous substances. The exposure assessment examines the transport and transformation of hazardous substances, in order to determine their environmental fate in media such as air, soil, and water. Models are used to estimate both the amount of hazardous substances reaching receptors and the form they take when doing so. In addition, the exposure assessment determines whether and how many persons are exposed (in the case of a human health assessment). If data are not available, it is necessary to make several reasonable assumptions in order to estimate actual exposure to target populations (Valaoras *et al.*, 1991).

For hazardous waste sites, this assessment involves an extensive review of each chemical identified as having an adverse health effect (target chemical), its point of release, the level, and to which environmental medium it is released. The extent and magnitude of environmental contamination is estimated by measuring chemical concentrations in specific environmental media. Analysis of exposed populations involves the identification, enumeration and characterisation of those population segments likely to be exposed. Finally, in an integrated exposure analysis, individual chemical-specific exposure estimates for each exposure route (inhalation, ingestion and dermal contact) are developed. For each exposed population, all exposures to each hazardous chemical are identified. Exposures are summed to integrate total exposure. The steps in exposure assessments at hazardous waste sites are shown below (Figure 21).

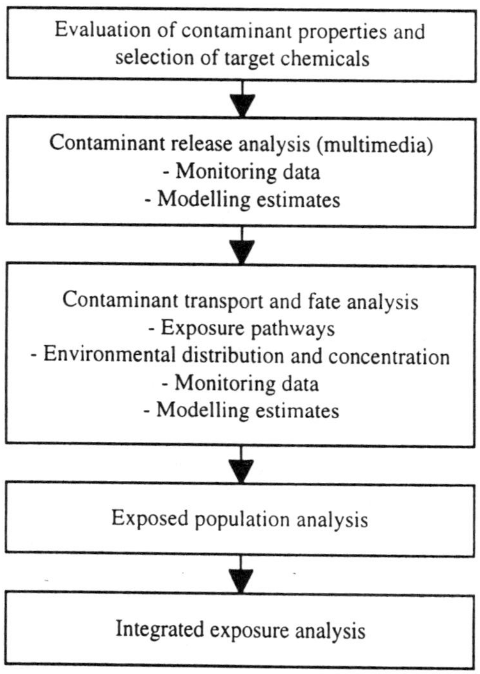


*Figure 21.* Elements of exposure assessment at hazardous waste sites (US EPA, 1988).

As shown in Figure 21, the risk assessment at a hazardous waste site can become quite complex, depending on the mixture of toxic substances identified in the vicinity of the site, and the amount of monitoring data needed for use in estimating exposure. Models of dispersion and transformation of substances in air, water and soil are necessary to supplement monitoring data, while the latter are used to validate the mathematical models.

Where sites are clearly identified with a private or public entity, the costs of sampling, risk assessment and remediation are borne by the responsible party. In the case of 'orphan' sites, the Superfund created out of legislation enacted in the 1980's is used to pay for these substantial costs.

The *risk characterisation* stage combines toxicity data from dose-response assessment with the exposure assessment, to reach conclusions on the total health risk. For carcinogenic substances, the risk assessment gives the probability of excess cancers occurring from the exposure that is estimated, stated as excess individual lifetime risks. Numerical estimates are usually accompanied by a discussion of the assumptions and uncertainties upon which they are based, since each risk assessment differs as to the weight of evidence for the hazard identification or the exposure assessment used to estimate risks. For non-cancer effects, the ratio of the reference dose to the lifetime average daily exposure gives an indication of the level of concern.

Certain limitations of risk assessment methodology should be noted before applying the process to estimate population risk. Although animal tests provide a systematic and quantifiable method of determining adverse health effects from exposure to toxic agents, they nevertheless involve uncertainty when transferring results from animals to humans. The uncertainty applies to the health effect itself, since different biological systems do not necessarily respond in identical ways. It also applies to the quantified level or dose that the animal test provides. Despite reasonable assumptions that are made to allow for body weight, metabolism, and other differences between the animal model and humans, there is incomplete understanding of the animal-to-human extrapolations for most adverse health effects.

Risk assessment is an evolving methodology, which is constantly being refined as scientific data becomes available. It has now been expanded to ecological risk assessment, and can identify a wide range of adverse health effects in humans as well as in animals and plants. Most environmental regulations dealing with hazardous wastes are implemented on the basis of this methodology.

## 3. Risk-Based Decision-Making

The regulation of toxic substances has been aided to a large extent by the ability of the scientific community to identify and measure the nature of chemical toxicity, and more importantly, by the development of quantitative risk assessment methods which can be consistently applied to estimate the risk to public health and the environment. There are thousands of toxic commercial chemicals and their by-products in the environment. Since it is not feasible to take regulatory action against all these substances, EPA seeks to develop a regulatory programme that achieves risk reduction across all environmental media for any given investment of resources. The regulatory programmes are adjusted to control most stringently the substances that produce the most risk. This is known as risk-based decision-making, a developing risk management tool which weighs the social costs of regulation and compares it to the benefits of risk reduction (Jennings and Valaoras, 1987).

Risk-based priority setting is also used at EPA's Office of Research and Development to select research projects. The goal is to focus research efforts on the greatest risk to human and environmental health. Comparative risk analysis is used to help identify the most pressing problems. A set of ecological and human health criteria are applied to potential areas of further research, including the following:

- have the problem's source(s) and risk been characterised sufficiently to develop risk management options?
- do risk management options exist (political, legal, socio-economic, technical)? If so, are they acceptable to stakeholders, implementable, reliable, and cost-effective?
- could new or improved technical solutions prevent or mitigate risk efficiently, cost-effectively, and in a manner acceptable to stakeholders?
- are other research organisations (e.g. agencies, industry) currently investigating, or developing, these solutions or interested in working in partnership?

Based on these criteria, and evaluating topics within each component of the risk paradigm (effects, exposure assessment, risk characterisation and risk management), priority is given to those projects which would make the greatest contribution to reducing uncertainty and improving risk management.

A further development of this process includes the modification of ecological risk assessment efforts from a traditional single-chemical, single-receptor approach to a more holistic, landscape-level ecological risk assessment. The Office of Research and Development is developing the ecological risk counterpart to the dose-response model used in human health risk assessment, designed to give managers a sense of ecosystem responses to various management alternatives.

## 4. Conclusions

Per capita waste generation in the US is double that of waste generated in western European countries. The US federal regulation of waste is based on quantitative risk assessments for hazardous waste. Such risk assessments are not performed on municipal solid waste, which accounts for roughly half of the waste stream, despite the fact that it contains household hazardous waste. Recycling and separation of hazardous substances from municipal waste streams are voluntary initiatives implemented at local level. EPA regulations based on risk assessments are used to prioritise actions, as well as to direct funding and research. The basic elements include a hazard identification, a dose-response assessment, exposure assessment and risk characterisation. This is combined with economic, social and political considerations to formulate risk management decisions. EPA uses extensive peer review to reach consensus on risk assessments, which are often subject to considerable debate, due to the uncertainties and interpretations which arise at each stage of the procedure. Today it has evolved into a sophisticated procedure which identifies many human health endpoints and can also be applied holistically to entire ecosystems on the basis of ecological risk assessment methodology.

## References

Jennings, A., and Valaoras, G. (1987) *Expected and Future Value of Risk; the Policy Implications of Quantitative Risk Analysis*, American Association for the Advancement of Science, 1987 Annual Meeting, Feb. 14-18, Chicago, Illinois.

National Research Council (NRC) (1983) Risk Assessment in the Federal Government: managing the process, Washington, D.C.

REHW (1998) Landfills are dangerous, *Rachel's Environment and Health Weekly* **#617**, September 24, http//www.rachel.org/.

United States Environmental Protection Agency (1986) A Survey of Household Hazardous Wastes and Related Collection Programs, EPA/530-SW-86-038, Washington, D.C.

US EPA - United States Environmental Protection Agency (1987) EPA Guidelines for Carcinogen Risk Assessment, Washington, D.C.

US EPA - United States Environmental Protection Agency (1988) Superfund Exposure Assessment Manual, EPA/540/1-88/001, Washington, D.C.

US EPA - United States Environmental Protection Agency (1998) US EPA Internet site http://www.epa.gov/epaoswer/osw/.

Valaoras, G., Cogliano, V., and Gibb, H. (1991) Risk assessment methodology applications in Greece: exposure to pesticides and chromium, in T. Lekkas (ed.) *Proceedings of the II Conference on Environmental Science and Technology*, Molyvos, Mytilene, Greece 2-5 September, 1991.

# HEALTH ISSUES ON WASTE MANAGEMENT

# BACKGROUND EXPOSURE TO DIOXINS AND PCB'S IN EUROPE AND THE RESULTING HEALTH EFFECTS

J.G. KOPPE
G. TEN TUSSCHER
P. DE BOER
*Neonatology Department*
*Emma Children's Hospital/Academic Medical Centre*
*University of Amsterdam*
*PO Box 22660*
*1100 DD Amsterdam*
*THE NETHERLANDS*

## Summary

The effect of exposure to background levels of dioxins and PCBs transplacentally and through breast-feeding on healthy new-born babies after an optimal pregnancy were studied in the Netherlands.

Negative effects were found on the development of the thyroid hormone metabolism, psychomotor development, behaviour and the immune system. Most of these effects were related to transplacental exposure. However, negative effects on the immune system and behaviour were related to current levels of PCBs measured in the blood of the child at the age of forty-two months. These findings can be extrapolated to areas in Europe with the same background levels.





*P. Nicolopoulou-Stamati et al. (eds.), Health Impacts of Waste Management Policies,* 135–154.
*Kluwer Academic Publishers. Printed in the Netherlands.*

## 1. Introduction

In 1977 Kees Olie and co-workers published an article on dioxins formed during municipal waste incineration and the emissions thereof into the environment (Olie *et al.*, 1977). During the early nineteen-eighties, Gunilla Lindström made known her discovery of dioxins in her own breast milk, and in breast milk of German mothers (Rappe *et al.*, 1986).

In 1986, dioxins were first detected in human breast milk, in the Netherlands, by Martin van den Berg *et al.* (1986). Following this, a world-wide survey on dioxin concentrations in human breast milk was conducted by the World Health Organisation (WHO, 1989).

The question raised was: What health consequences these dioxin levels could have for a population? In order to address this issue studies were begun in the Netherlands in 1987 and in 1990 (Koppe *et al.*, 1988; Koopman-Esseboom, 1995; Huisman, 1996).

In animal studies, dioxin exposure has been demonstrated to have effects on various homeostatic systems. One of the most sensitive systems affected was the immune system. At body burdens of only 5 ng TEQ/kg body weight (toxic equivalency factor per kilogram) effects on the immune system were elicited in non-human primates (De Vito *et al.*, 1995).

In addition, it became clear that the foetus and the new-born baby are the most vulnerable subjects. Their developing systems are exposed to the dioxin concentrations in the mothers womb during pregnancy, and post-natally through ingestion of highly polluted breast milk.

The vulnerability of the foetus and the new-born is the result of the many imprinting processes that take place in the perinatal period (Csaba, 1991). For example, for human beings it is known that the imprinting of the sexual identity takes place in the second and third trimester of pregnancy, in response to hormone production. Not only does genetic determination play a decisive role in sexual development, but environmental factors do, too.

Another aspect of imprinting is hormonal and enzymal imprinting. Faulty imprinting caused by the introduction of certain hormones, or chemicals mimicking these hormones, during the sensitive period, can cause disturbances in homeostasis. For instance, the setpoint (the optimal concentration point) of the thyroid hormonal system could be set (slightly) higher or lower. A lowering of the setpoint for body temperature was detected in rats exposed to dioxins during the perinatal period (Gordon *et al.*, 1995).

The setpoint for the induction of enzymes can also be altered, as can be seen in the alteration in the activity of the cytochrome P-450 system. The activity of this enzyme system, responsible for de-toxification, may be altered in a positive or negative way in response to prolonged periods of exposure to toxins. In rat studies, Benzo(a)pyrene has been shown to change this activity setpoint, resulting in a delay of enzyme induction (Csaba *et al.*, 1987). This may be an ominous sign in the development of malignancies. A delay in enzyme induction may mean longer exposure to toxic chemicals, or to toxic chemical metabolites, possibly resulting in disadvantageous health effects.

Behavioural imprinting is another example in which environmental influences in the perinatal period play a pertinent role. Appropriate reactions are dependent on appropriately working hormone systems in a baby.

A well-known example of imprinting is that of the immune system in the perinatal period and during infancy.

In all four of the above-mentioned fields, sexual, hormonal, enzymal and behavioural, abnormalities can be expected, and have been elicited, in relation to exposure to chemicals such as dioxins and polychlorinated biphenyls (PCBs).

It is not only true that the effects on imprinting may be hazardous, but also that the direct effects of chemicals and pharmaceuticals used by the mother may be detrimental; an example of such a pharmaceutical is the maternal usage of anticonvulsants. Interestingly enough, an important part of the PCBs detected in human breast milk are phenobarbital-like, e.g. the PCB congeners -138, -153, -180.

Let us now consider both the direct causal effects and the effects of faulty imprinting in human babies, and their follow-up, in the light of the current background levels of dioxins and PCBs.

## 2. Direct Effects

### *2.1. Vitamin K Metabolism*

Analogous to the effects of phenobarbital, it was hypothesised that PCBs and dioxins can disturb vitamin K metabolism in utero and after birth, resulting in a deficiency of the vitamin (Koppe *et al.*, 1989).

Vitamin K is necessary for the carboxylation of prothrombin in the liver, and is probably also used for similar reactions elsewhere in the body.

In human babies a new disease entity has been described by Lane: the late haemorrhagic disease of the new-born (HDN). HDN is based on vitamin K deficiency and is characterised by severe intracranial bleeding between one and three months after birth (Lane and Hathaway, 1985).

Like dioxins, and dioxin-like PCBs, ortho-substituted non-planar PCBs are commonly encountered, and can be found in rather high concentrations in breast milk - 63 per cent of the total amount of PCBs in human breast milk is ortho-substituted non-planar PCB-22, -52, -138, -153 and -180. These PCBs have phenobarbital-like effects. They are capable of inducing enzymes in the liver, resulting in increased vitamin K metabolism, which may ultimately lead to deficiency of the vitamin. These effects have been shown in animal studies. In addition, vitamin K deficient haemorrhagic states were more prevalent in male animals - as this state is counteracted by oestrogen. Pre-treatment of female rats with androgen decreased prothrombin levels, resulting in an increased incidence of the vitamin K deficiency haemorrhagic state.

Three forms of HDN are described: the early, the classic and the late form. The early form can result in a life-threatening haemorrhage during pregnancy, during delivery or within

24 hours after birth. This is known to occur in conjunction with maternal usage of anticonvulsant medication, certain antibiotics, and tuberculostatics - all potent inducers of the hepatic cytochrome P-450 enzyme complex.

The classic form involves exclusively breastfed infants, occurs during the first seven days of life and results mostly in a benign gastro-intestinal bleeding, the so-called 'melaena neonatorum'. Since the discovery of the role of vitamin K, the vitamin has been shown to be an effective treatment for babies exhibiting melaena during the first neonatal week.
The late form of HDN, in contrast to the early and classic form, is a new disease entity. It is characterised by severe intracranial bleeding between one and three months after birth. It is found exclusively in breastfed children not receiving extra vitamin K supplementation.

Epidemics of this disease have been described. In Japan, in particular, four hundred and twenty-five cases of late vitamin K deficiency bleeding occurred between 1981 and 1985, including two hundred and eighty-four males and one hundred and forty-one females. Once again a preponderance of males (Nagao and Nakayama, 1984). In Germany, Holland and England sporadic cases of late HDN have been described since 1980 (Koppe *et al.*, 1989). Furthermore, in a Dutch study about ten per cent of breastfed babies had biochemical abnormalities in their blood indicating a vitamin K deficient state (Widdershoven, 1987). These babies had not received extra vitamin K supplementation after birth. Vitamin K levels are normally low during pregnancy and after birth. As a result of efficient recycling only nanograms of vitamin K are needed per day (Pietersma-de Bruyn *et al.*, 1990). A breastfed infant receives about 5 micrograms per day of the vitamin - 1000 times more than it needs. However, when the cytochrome P-450 enzyme complex is activated, vitamin K is metabolised and excreted with the bile, and this may rapidly lead to a state of deficiency in an exclusively breastfed baby. Activation of this enzyme complex in the perinatal period is thus a toxic phenomenon.

Extra vitamin K supplementation is therefore used in Europe today in order to prevent vitamin K deficiency during breastfeeding. Intramuscular injections of milligrams of vitamin K are sufficiently effective in the prevention of bleeding. However a relation between leukaemia and intramuscular vitamin K injections has been elicited, in epidemiological studies, so that oral supplementation is now recommended (Golding *et al.*, 1990). Why nature chooses to keep vitamin K levels low in babies is unknown. An explanation might lie in the endocrine-disrupting properties of the menadione molecule, a synthetic form of vitamin K, which has inherently oestrogenic properties (Mukerjée, 1997; Bouwman, 1994).

### 2.2. Congenital Anomalies

Infants with congenital PCB poisoning in Taiwan were characterised by hyperpigmentation, intra-uterine growth retardation, natal teeth, pigmented dysplasia of the nails, hirsutism, hypertelorism, conjunctivitis, clinodactyly, widely open fontanelles and spotty calcifications of the skull. Mortality was high, with 25 per cent of these hyperpigmented babies dying within four years of birth. Respiratory distress and pneumonia during the first six months of life was common (Rogan *et al.*, 1988).

In the discussion of what effects may be expected as a result of the background levels of PCBs and dioxins, congenital anomalies did not have the highest priority. Animal studies have shown that the doses of toxic chemicals have to be rather high in order to cause malformations. In Europe this resulted in studies on this toxicological aspect being neglected, possibly wrongly so. In certain regions where exposure is high, clusters of defects can be found. In a literature search, several publications indicate congenital defects, for instance, amongst inhabitants in the neighbourhood of landfills, or after the spraying of insecticides (Dolk *et al.*, 1998; White *et al.*, 1988). Additionally, the open incineration of chemicals may cause an increase in congenital malformations as described in these proceedings (ten Tusscher *et al.*, 1998).

After the Seveso incident, no increased incidence of congenital malformations was detected. However, many women underwent abortions after the disaster, for fear of the consequences for their unborn baby (Mastroiacovo *et al.*, 1988).

What is striking in all the publications relating PCBs, dioxins, insecticides and herbicides with the incidence of congenital malformations is the reported increased incidence of midline defects. This same increased incidence in midline defects is seen with maternal usage of anticonvulsant medication during pregnancy (Koppe *et al.*, 1973). Cleft lip and/or palate, spina bifida, gastroschisis, heart defects, hypospadias and inguinal hernias are amongst the malformations mentioned: all are examples of midline defects (ten Tusscher *et al.*, 1998; Koppe *et al.*, 1973; Gordon and Shy, 1981; Nelson *et al.*, 1979).

Presently, the incidence of hypospadias, both in Europe and the United States, is rising. Endocrine-disrupting chemicals with oestrogenic or anti-androgenic effects are blamed for this rise (Dolk, 1998; Paulozzi *et al.*, 1997).

Another so far unexplained finding is the fact that parents with high levels of TCDD after the Seveso incident gave birth almost exclusively to female offspring (Mocarelli *et al.*, 1996).

### *2.3. Thyroid Hormone Levels*

Dioxins and dibenzofurans have a similar chemical structure to that of thyroid hormones (Figure 22). Structurally, the only difference is that the chlorine atom of the former is situated in the position of the iodine atom of thyroxin. This structural similarity gave rise to the hypothesis that dioxins and furans are able to mimic the working of thyroxin, and while this effect has long been suspected, it has never been proven (Rozman *et al.*, 1984; Rozman *et al.*, 1985).

During human gestation, the human foetal hypothalamic-pituitary-thyroid system is relatively quiescent and foetal thyroid hormone production is limited until a gestational age of eighteen to twenty weeks. During the second half of gestation, the functioning of the foetal thyroid gland increases, under the influence of an increasing Thyroid Stimulating Hormone (TSH) concentration. There is also a progressive increase in the concentration ratio of free $T_4$ to TSH, suggesting maturation of the hypothalamic-pituitary negative feedback control system for TSH secretion. *'Thyroid system maturation during the latter half of gestation can be characterised as a balance among increasing hypothalamic Thyrotropic Releasing Hormone (TRH)-secretion, increasing pituitary sensitivity to thyroid hormone inhibition of TSH release, and increasing thyroid follicular cell sensitivity to TSH'*, according to Fisher (1998). Chemicals mimicking thyroid hormones can disturb this process. In this light, studies on the effects of background exposure to dioxins in our country also focused on the thyroid hormone metabolism. In both the Zaandam study of Pluim (1993) and the Rotterdam study of Koopman-Esseboom *et al.*

(1994), abnormalities in thyroid hormone metabolism were detected in relation to dioxin levels. Pluim (1993) detected a significantly higher $T_4$ concentration during the first eleven weeks of life in the higher-exposed babies, whom also exhibited a significantly higher TSH concentration at eleven weeks of age.

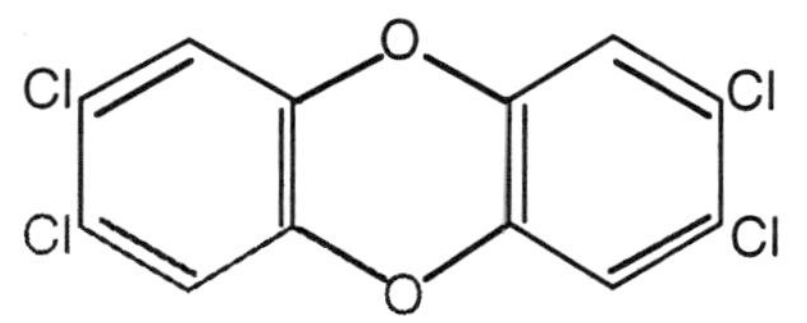


2,3,7,8 dibenzo-p-dioxin

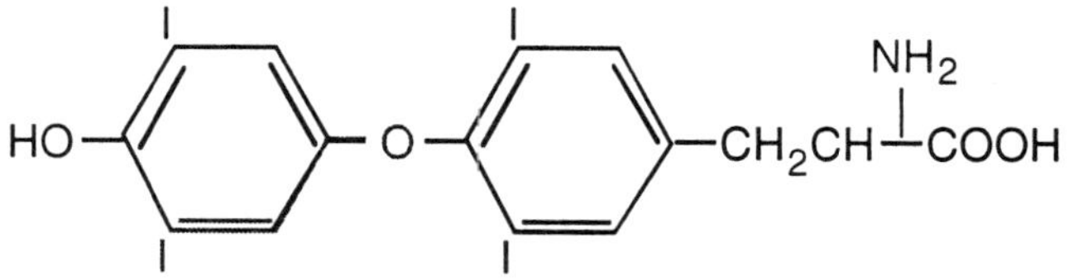


3,5,3',5'-tetraiodothyronine (thyroxine[$T_4$])

*Figure 22.* Chemical structure of 2,3,7,8 dibenzo-p-dioxin and 3,5,3',5' tetraiodothyronine. Note the structural similarity between the parts indicated in grey.

Koopman-Esseboom *et al.* (1994) detected lower free thyroxin ($FT_4$) and $T_4$ concentrations shortly after birth, and also higher TSH concentrations at two weeks and three months of age in her higher exposure group. In her study, she found no relation between dioxin levels in the neonatal period and neurological abnormalities, and no relation between the lower thyroxin concentrations in the neonatal period and neurological abnormalities (Koopman-Esseboom *et al.*, 1997).

Thyroid hormones also play a part in brown adipose tissue thermogenesis. This form of heat production involves the rapid burning of the triglycerides that are packaged around the great vessels, in order to keep the baby warm. From animal studies it is known that this manner of thermogenesis, through the burning of brown adipose tissue, is jeopardised by dioxins, making survival after birth more difficult.

## 2.4. *White Blood Cells and Blood Platelets*

Pluim (1993) detected lower concentrations of granulocytes and monocytes on the seventh day of life in the prenatally higher dioxin-exposed babies. At eleven weeks of age the concentration of blood platelets were lower in relation to the amount of dioxin the babies ingested with their breast milk. In Rotterdam a similar decrease, in relation to pre- and postnatal exposure to dioxins, was detected in the concentration of granulocytes at three months of age, together with a lower monocyte count. The lowering of white blood cell and blood platelet counts is probably due to an inhibition of the bone marrow by dioxins. In the follow-up study after approximately two years, both studies discovered that the exhibited lowering of these white blood cells was no longer evident (Weisglas-Kuperus *et al.*, 1995; Ilsen *et al.*, 1996). An extensive reduction of lymphocyte stem cells was seen in the bone marrow of the offspring of maternal rats treated with one dose of dioxins of 10 microgram per kilogram body weight during pregnancy (Fine *et al.*, 1988). Another study in non-human primates showed a lowering of CD4+ lymphocytes and an increase in CD8+ lymphocytes after a single dose of only 10 nanograms TCDD per kilogram body weight (Neubert *et al.*, 1990). Thus, direct effects on the immune system, in those of humans too, are already seen at low background exposure levels.

## 2.5. *Infectious Diseases in Infancy*

In follow-up studies no significant differences in the number or sort of infectious diseases were detected, up to the age of about two years (Weisglas-Kuperus *et al.*, 1995; Ilsen *et al.*, 1996). Yet, in the Rotterdam study, at the age of forty-two months more middle-ear infections were found in relation to the current PCB-levels of the children (Patandin, 1999). This relation to the current PCB-levels, however, might not be related to a disturbed immunological function, but rather could be a direct effect of PCBs on the epithelium of the Eustachian tube. It is known that PCB-metabolites preferentially accumulate in the Clara cells of the lung, resulting in hypersecretion. Due to the fact that the epithelium of the lung is of the same origin as that of the Eustachian tube (which, for instance, also produces surfactant), it is logical to offer the hypersecretion in the Eustachian tube as an explanation for the middle-ear infections (Lund *et al.*, 1985). This hypersecretion could also be an explanation for the increase in respiratory diseases seen after PCB poisoning (Shigematsu *et al.*, 1978).

The afore-mentioned studies were conducted amongst normal, healthy, pregnant mothers and their babies. Pathology in the mothers and babies, or complications during pregnancy, delivery, or in the neonatal period, led to the exclusion of the subjects from the particular study. This approach has the disadvantage that toxic effects resulting in disease during pregnancy, delivery or in the neonatal period are not detected. For instance, infections, haemorrhaging and new disease entities may not be detected due to the exclusion of the subjects from the studies.

Another new disease entity in the new-born, apart from late HDN, is the group B streptococcus epidemic. This epidemic has its unexplained origin in the sixties (Gerards, 1985). It can be hypothesised that this rise in group B streptococcus infections is related to background PCB and dioxin exposure. A study in the modulation in serum complement levels following dioxin exposure in mice has been published. The dioxins enhanced the susceptibility of the mice to *Streptococcus pneumoniae,* a bacterial pathogen. The host defence is complement-mediated in mice. Humans also rely on their complement system to combat this bacterial pathogen (White *et al.*, 1986). The complement system of the human new-born is deficient, rendering the infant susceptible to infections. This is not so for the mother and it is unknown why streptococci infest her cervix during pregnancy, leading to premature delivery and to severely ill babies infected in utero or during delivery. In order that this hypothesis can be studied, ill babies in particular must be involved, making the study inherently more difficult to carry out.

### 2.6. Birthweight and Growth

The offspring of mothers accidentally exposed to PCBs and furans during pregnancy are characterised by low birthweights (Rogan *et al.*, 1988). Reduced birthweights and smaller head circumferences are also described in the study of the babies of mothers who consumed fish from Lake Michigan (Fein *et al.*, 1984). In follow-up studies, the children remained smaller than their contemporaries and there was no catch-up growth (Jacobson *et al.*, 1990; Guo *et al.*, 1994). The wives of fishermen from the east coast of Sweden known to have consumed PCB- and dioxin-polluted fish from the Baltic Sea gave birth to children with lower birthweights than their counterparts from the west coast (Rylander *et al.*, 1995).

In Rotterdam, effects on birthweight and reduced growth up to three months of age were also found in relation to the sum of PCBs in cord blood and in maternal plasma. The PCB congeners 118, 138, 153 and 180 - most of which are phenobarbital-like - were detected. This is in accordance with studies of the children of mothers using phenobarbital, in which lower birthweights are also described (Seip, 1976). It is a very sobering and worrying thought that the levels of these PCBs are so high that they have an effect on birthweight. The reduction in birthweight is approximately 90 g in the group with median PCB levels of 0.41 g/L in cord plasma. This means that an infant with a cord PCB level above the P90 (i.e. two standard deviations above the median), and therefore having a PCB level of 0.80 g/l, has a birthweight of 165 g less than that of an infant at the P10 level (Patandin, 1999). Thus, even at background levels found in Europe, effects on birthweight and growth are obvious.

In the Zaandam study, liver size was measured by means of ultrasound. As related to the perinatal dioxin exposure, an increase in hepatic size was expected, contrary to the trend towards a smaller size found at two weeks of age. Between two and eleven weeks of age, the liver increased in size, more so in the higher-exposed babies than the lower, and was the same for the two groups by eleven weeks of age (Pluim, 1993).

## 3. Effects of Faulty Imprinting

During the critical perinatal period, environmental influences like dioxins and PCBs can disturb hormonal and enzymal activity setpoints. This may result in functional developmental disabilities in later life. During the first trimester all neurones in the brain are formed. Yet, it is during the second and third trimester, especially around thirty weeks gestational age, that the growth and development of the brain takes place, characterised by the forming of dendrites, connecting the neurones, and by the start of glial myelinisation.

Structures in the brain necessary to process visual and auditory signals, for instance for language development, are then formed. This process proceeds, albeit somewhat slower than prenatally, during the first year of life, and slower still up to adolescence.

During pregnancy, the developmental process depends largely on hormones. For instance, testosterone is necessary around the thirtieth week of pregnancy for the typical male brain development, characterised by good visuo-spatial abilities. Lowering of the testosterone levels, for example as a result of an enhanced prenatal liver metabolism, causes impairment of visuo-spatial abilities later in life (Dessens, 1996). This is seen in the children of mothers using anticonvulsant medication during pregnancy. Therefore, long-term follow-up studies are essential in order to effectively relate background exposure in the perinatal period to later health effects.

### *3.1. Psychomotor Development*

In a study carried-out in North Carolina, hypotonia and hyporeflexia in relation to prenatal exposure to PCBs were already detected in the neonatal period, shortly after birth (Rogan *et al.*, 1986). During infancy the higher-exposed children exhibited developmental delays in gross motor function (Gladen *et al.*, 1988). In the children of mothers ingesting PCB-polluted fish from Lake Michigan a poorer visual recognition memory (Fagan Test) was associated with increasing prenatal PCB exposure. The levels of PCBs in the study in Michigan were only slightly above US background levels and comparable with Dutch levels.

The Zaandam group was studied at the age of two years and seven months. Signs of enhanced neuromotor maturation were found and it was hypothesised that this may be due to the thyroxin-antagonistic action of dioxins (Ilsen *et al.*, 1996).

The Rotterdam and Groningen group of children were studied at one year and six months, and at three years and six months. At one year and six months, the neuromotor development was negatively related to the sum of the transplacental PCB exposure. The congeners 118, 138, 153 and 180 were measured - most of these PCBs are phenobarbital-like (Huisman *et al.*, 1995). A negative relation was once again found with cognitive functioning and the sum of the phenobarbital-like PCBs measured in cord blood, at three years and six months of age (Patandin, 1999). Overall cognitive functioning was negatively influenced, as was the verbal comprehension score. This finding is in accordance with the study of the Jacobson's, who noted a negative effect of prenatal exposure to PCBs on cognitive functioning, at the age of four years (Jacobson *et al.*, 1990). Furthermore, at the age of eleven years, IQ-test scores were lower in the higher-exposed children. Difficulties in verbal comprehension were elicited and the ability to concentrate was reduced in the higher-exposed children. The latter were more than twice as likely to be two years behind in reading skills and word comprehension (Jacobson and Jacobson, 1996).

Similar attention and verbal IQ problems have been detected in children prenatally exposed to anticonvulsants. Negative effect on psycho-sexual development and reproductive performance were also detected in the latter group (Dessens, 1996).

Long-term follow-up studies, into and throughout adulthood, are necessary in order to detect abnormalities in sensitive endpoints like psycho-sexual development and reproductive performance.

### *3.2. Behaviour*

Prenatal exposure to PCBs and furans was associated with negative behavioural effects amongst the intoxicated Yusho offspring. The children were apathetic and indifferent (Harada, 1976). Monkeys exposed prenatally to PCBs exhibited hyperactive behaviour during infancy. This was followed by inactivity at four years of age (Bowman and Heironimus, 1981). The children of fish-eating mothers from Lake Michigan displayed reduced activity, with current body burdens of PCBs, at four years of age.

In the Rotterdam study, hyperactivity and slower mean reaction times were detected in relation to the current PCB-levels in the children at forty-two months of age. Attention during free play behaviour was reduçed relative to cord and maternal PCB exposure (Patandin, 1999).

Thus, we once again see that both prenatal and postnatal PCB exposure have a detrimental influence on behaviour.

### *3.3. Immune System*

We have already looked at the direct effects on white blood cells *(vide supra)*. There are also subtle signs that the leucocytes may be influenced through faulty imprinting during the critical perinatal period. Weisglas-Kuperus *et al.* (1995) published their findings on low-level prenatal exposure to PCDD's and PCBs in their Rotterdam group: this exposure may influence the development of particular immune cell populations. Eighteen-month-old children exhibited an increase in T cells (CD8+, amongst others) which persisted until the age of forty-two months. However, at forty-two months the increase was related to the sum of maternal PCBs and not to the I-TEQ dioxin (Patandin, 1999). Additionally, amongst the forty-two-month-old children, a higher incidence of chickenpox was noted relative to the sum of the maternal PCBs, and levels of antibodies to measles were lower in relation to the sum of the PCB levels in cord blood (Patandin, 1999). It remains unclear why the relationships are found with different exposures: some PCBs, others dioxins. Possibly the TEQ-concept is not a suitable or not sensitive (enough) method for the endpoints studied. The fact that the relationship was later found with PCBs, and not with dioxins, does not eliminate the exposure to dioxins as a cause.

## 4. Conclusions

In studies of human beings effects from exposure to background levels of PCBs and dioxins in the Netherlands have been found.

Negative effects on immunity, psychomotor development and behaviour have been found, relative to dioxin exposure, expressed with help of the TEQ-concept. The effects, relative to the sum of the PCBs, as measured in the plasma of the mother during her pregnancy, in the cord blood at birth, and with the current PCB-levels, are respectively: neuromotor functioning, cognitive functioning and behaviour, and immunity and middle-ear infections. The PCBs noted are mostly phenobarbital-like (congeners 118, 138, 153, 180). Using the TEQ-concept to measure the amount of dioxins and dioxin-like PCBs may not be suitable for the endpoints studied. Is the exposure to the phenobarbital-like PCBs more important? The relation found with these phenobarbital-like PCBs is probably a causal relationship, the more so because of what we know about the effects on humans of phenobarbital itself. However, dioxins cannot be excluded as a cause and might very well play a role as well, which may become evident if another method to measure dioxin toxicity is used. Finally, it is also possible that dioxin-exposure is related to other (as yet unstudied) endpoints.

## References

Bouwman, C.A. (1994) Modulation of Vitamin K dependent blood coagulation by chlorinated biphenyls and dioxins in rats, Thesis, Universiteit Utrecht, The Netherlands, ISBN: 90-393-0581-1.

Bowman, R.E., and Heironimus, M.P. (1981) Hypoactivity in adolescent monkeys perinatally exposed to PCBs and hyperactive as juveniles, *Neurobehav. Toxicol. Teratol.* **3**, 15-18.

Csaba, G., Bobozy, O., and Szeberényi, Sz. (1987) A single neonatal treatment with methylcholanthrene of benzo(a)pyrene alters microsomal enzyme activity for life, *Acta Phys. Hung.* **70**, 87-91.

Csaba G. (1991) Interactions between the Genetic Programme and Environmental Influences in the Perinatal Critical Period, *Zoölogical Science* **8**, 813-825.

De Vito, M.J., Birnbaum, L.S., Farland, W.H., and Gasiewicz, T.A. (1995) Comparisons of estimated human body burdens of dioxinlike chemicals and TCDD body burdens in experimentally exposed animals, *Environmental Health Perspectives* **103 (9)**, 820-830.

Dessens, A.B. (1996) Prenatal exposure to phenobarbital and diphantoïn: a study on long-lasting consequences, Thesis, University of Amsterdam, The Netherlands.

Dolk, H. (1998) Rise in prevalence of hypospadias, *Lancet* **351**, 770.

Dolk, H., Vrijheid, M., Armstrong, B., Abramsky, L., Bianchi, F., Garne, E., Nelen, V., Robert, E., Scott, J.E.S., Stone, D., and Tenconi, R. (1998) Risk of congenital anomalies near hazardous-waste landfill sites in Europe: the Eurohazcon study, *Lancet* **352**, August 8.

Fein, G.G., Jacobson, J.L., Jacobson, S.W., Schwartz, P.M., and Dowler, J.K. (1984) Prenatal exposure to polychlorinated biphenyls: effects on birth size and gestational age, *J. Pediatr.* **105**, 315-320.

Fine, J.S., Gasiewicz, T.A., and Silverstone, A.E. (1988) Lymphocyte Stem Cell Alterations following Perinatal Exposure to 2,3,7,8-Tetrachlorodibenzo-p-dioxin, *Molecular Pharmacology* **35**, 18-25.

Fisher, D.A. (1998) The thyroïd function in premature infants, *Clinics in Perinatology* **25** **(4)**, 999-1014.

Gerards, L.J. (1985) Group B streptococci in the perinatal period, PhD thesis, University of Utrecht, The Netherlands.

Gladen, B.C., Rogan, W.J., Hardy, P., Thullen, J., Tingelstad, J., and Tully, M. (1988) Development after exposure to polychlorinated biphenyls and dichlorodiphenyl transplacentally and through human milk, *J. Pediatr.* **113**, 991-995.

Golding, J., Paterson, M., and Kinlen, L.J. (1990) Factors associated with childhood cancer in a national cohort study, *Br. J. Cancer* **62**, 304-308.

Gordon, J.E., and Shy, C.M. (1981) Agricultural chemical use and congenital cleft lip and/or palate, *Arch. Environ. Health* **36**, 213-221.

Gordon, C.J., Gray, Jr. L.E., and Monteiro-Rivière, N.A. (1995) Temperature regulation and metabolism in rats exposed perinatally to dioxin: Permanent change in regulated body temperature, *Toxicol. Appl. Pharmacol.* **133**, 172-176.

Guo, Y.L., Lin, C.J., Yao, W.J., Ryan, J.J., and Hsu, C.C. (1994) Musculoskeletal changes in children prenatally exposed to polychlorinated biphenyls and related compounds (Yu-Cheng children), *J. Toxicol. Environ. Health* **41**, 93.

Harada, M. (1976) Intra-uterine poisoning. Clinical and Epidemiological studies and significance of the problem, *Bull. Inst. Const. Med. Kumamoto University* **25** **(Suppl.)**, 1-69.

Huisman, M., Koopman-Esseboom, C., Lanting, C.I., vanderPaauw, C.G., Tuinstra, L., Fidler, V., Weisglas-Kuperus, N., Sauer, P.J.J., Boersma, E.R., and Touwen, B.C.L. (1995) Neurological condition in 18-month-old children perinatally exposed to polychlorinated biphenyls and dioxins, *Early Human Development* **43**, 165-176.

Huisman, M. ( 1996) Effects of early infant nutrition and perinatal exposure to PCBs and dioxins on neurological development. A study of breast-fed and formula-fed infants, Thesis, Rijksuniversiteit Groningen, The Netherlands.

Ilsen, A., Briët, J.M., Koppe, J.G., Pluim, H.J., and Oosting, J. (1996) Signs of enhanced neuromotor maturation in children due to perinatal load with background levels of dioxins, *Chemosfere* **33** **(7)**, 1317-1326.

Jacobson, J.L., Jacobson, S.W., and Humphrey, H.E. (1990) Effects of exposure to PCBs and related compounds on growth and activity in children, *Neurotoxicol. Teratol.* **12**, 319-326.

Jacobson, J.L., and Jacobson, S. (1996) Intellectual impairment in children exposed to polychlorinated biphenyls in utero, *N. Engl. J. Med.* **335 (11)**, 783-789.

Koopman-Esseboom, C., Morse, D.C., Weisglas-Kuperus, N., Lutkeschipholt, IJ., Vanderpaauw, C.G., and Tuinstra, L.G. (1994) Effects of dioxins and polychlorinated biphenyls on thyroïd hormone status of pregnant women and their infants, *Pediatr. Research* **36 (4)**, 468-473.

Koopman-Esseboom, C. (1995) Effects of Perinatal exposure to PCBs and dioxins on early human development, Thesis, Erasmus University, Rotterdam, The Netherlands.

Koopman-Esseboom, C., Huisman, M., Touwen, B.C.L., Brouwer, A., Sauer, P.J.J., and Weisglas-Kuperus, N. (1997) Newborn infants diagnosed as neurological abnormal with relation to PCB and dioxin exposure and their thyroïd-hormone status, *Dev. Med. Child. Neurol.* **39 (11)**, 785.

Koppe, J.G., Bosman, W., Oppers, V.M., Spaans, F., and Kloosterman, G.J. (1973) Epilepsie en aangeboren afwijkingen, *Ned. T. Geneesk.* **117 (6)**, 220-224. (in Dutch)

Koppe, J.G., Pluim, H.J., and Olie, K. (1988) Breast milk, PCBs, Dioxins and Vitamin K deficiency, in L. Stern (ed.) *Physiologic Foundations of Perinatal Care*, Elsevier, Amsterdam, pp. 115-131.

Koppe, J.G., Pluim, H.J., and Olie, K. (1989) Breast milk, PCBs, dioxins and vitamin K deficiency, *J. Royal Soc. Of Med.* **82**, 416-420.

Lane, P., and Hathaway, W.E. (1985) Vitamin K in infancy, *J. Ped.* **106**, 351-361.

Lund, J., Brandt, I., Andersson, O., Poellinger, L., and Gustafsson, J.-A. (1985) In vitro characterisation of possible mechanisms underlying the selective in vivo accumulation of the PCB metabolite 4,4'-bis (methylsulphonyl)-2,2',5,5'-tetrachlorobiphenyl in the lung, *Molec. Pharmacol.* **27**, 314.

Mastroiacovo, P., Spagnolo, A., Mani, E., Meazza, L., Bertollini, R., and Segni, G. (1988) Birth defects in the Seveso Artea After TCDD Contamination, *JAMA* **259 (11)**, 1668-1672.

Mocarelli, P., Brambilla, P., Gerthoux, P.M., Patterson, D.G., Needham, L.L. (1996) Change in sex ratio with exposure to dioxin, Letter, *Lancet* **348 (9024)**, 409.

Mukerjée, D. (1997) Rationale for considering neurotoxic activities of ortho-substituted non-planar PCBs in risk assessment, *Organohalogen Compounds* **34**, 145-149.

Nagao, T., and Nakayama, K. (1984) Vitamin K deficiency in infancy in Japan, *Pediatrics* **74**, 315-316.

Nelson, C.J., Holson, J.F., and Green, H.G. (1979) Retrospective study of the relationship between agricultural use of 2,4,5-T and cleft palate occurrence in Arkansas, *Teratology* **19**, 377-384.

Neubert, R., Jacob-Müller, U., Stahlmann, R., Helge, H., and Neubert, D. (1990) Polyhalogenated dibenzo-p-dioxins and the immune system, *Arch. Toxicol.* **64**, 345-349.

Olie, K., Vermeulen, P.L., and Hutzinger, O. (1977) Chlorodibenzo-p-dioxins and chlorodibenzofurans are trace components of fly and flue gas of some municipal incinerators in the Netherlands, *Chemosfere* **6**, 455-459.

Patandin, S. (1999) Effects of environmental exposure to polychlorinated biphenyls and dioxins on growth and development in young children, PhD thesis, Erasmus University, Rotterdam, The Netherlands.

Paulozzi, L.J., Erickson, J.D., and Jackson, R.J. (1997) Hypospadias trends in two US surveillance systems, *Pediatrics* **100**, 831-834.

Pietersma-de Bruyn, A.L.J.M., van der Haard, P.M.M., Beunis, M.H., Hamulyak, K., and Kuijpers, J.C. (1990) Vitamin K levels and coagulation factors in healthy term newborns till 4 weeks after birth, *Haemostasis* **20**, 8-14.

Pluim, H.J. (1993) Dioxins. Pre- and postnatal exposure in the human newborn, PhD thesis, University of Amsterdam, The Netherlands.

Rappe, C., Nygrèn, M., Lindström, G., and Hansson, M. (1986) Dioxins and dibenzofurans in blood and adipose tissue of European origin, *Chemosfere* **15**, 1635-1639.

Rogan, W.J., Gladen, B.C., and McKinney, J.D. (1986) Neonatal effects of transplacental exposure to PCBs and DDE, *J. Pediatr.* **109 (113)**, 335-341.

Rogan, W.J., Gladen, B.C., Kun-Long Hung, Shin-Lan Koong, Ling-Yu Shih, Taylor, J.S., Ying-Chin Wu, Yang, D., Ragan, N.B., and Chen-Chin Hsu (1988) Congenital Poisoning by Polychlorinated Biphenyls and their contaminants in Taiwan, *Science* **241**, 334-336.

Rozman, K., Rozman, T., and Greim, H. (1984) Effect of thyroïdectomy and thyroxin on 2,3,7,8-tetrachlorodibenzo-p-dioxin (TCDD) induced toxicity, *Toxicol. Appl. Pharmacol.* **72**, 372.

Rozman, K., Rozman, T., Scheufler, E., Pazdernik, T., and Greim, H. (1985) Thyroïd hormones modulate the toxicity of 2,3,7,8-tetrachlorodibenzo-p-dioxin (TCDD), *J. Toxicol. Environ. Health* **16**, 481.

Rylander, L., Strömberg, U., and Hagmar, L. (1995) Decreased birthweight among infants born to women with a high dietary intake of fish contaminated with persistent organochlorine compounds, *Scand. J. Work Environ. Health* **21**, 368.

Seip, M. (1976) Growth retardation, dysmorphic facies and minor malformations following massive exposure to phenobarbitone in utero, *Acta Paed. Scand.* **65**, 617-621.

Shigematsu, N., Ishimaru, S., Saito, R., Ikeda, R.T., Sugiyama, K., and Masuda, Y. (1978) Respiratory involvement in polychlorinated biphenyl poisoning, *Environ. Res.* **16**, 92-100.

ten Tusscher, G.W., Stam, G., and Koppe, J.G. (1998). Open chemical combustions resulting in a local increased incidence of orofacial clefts, *Organohalogen Compounds* **37**, 337-340.

Van den Berg, M., Van der Wielen, F.W.M., Olie, K., and Van Boxtel, C.J. (1986) The presence of PCDD's and PCDF's in human breast milk from the Netherlands, *Chemosfere* **15**, 693-706.

Weisglas-Kuperus, N., Sas, T.C.J., Koopman-Esseboom, C., Vanderzwan, C.W., Deridder, M.A.J., Beishuizen, A., Hooijkaas, H., and Sauer, P.J.J. (1995) Immunologic effects of background prenatal and postnatal exposure to dioxins and polychlorinated biphenyls in dutch infants, *Pediatric Research* **38** **(3)**, 404-410.

White, K.L., Lysy, H.H., Ann McCay, J., and Anderson, A. (1986) Modulation of serum complement levels following exposure to polychlorinated dibenzo-p-dioxins, *Toxicol. Appl. Pharmacol.* **84**, 209-219.

White, F.M.M., Cohen, F.G., Sherman, G., and McCurdy, R. (1988) Chemicals, birth defects and still-births in New Brunswick: associations with agricultural activity, *CMAJ* **138**, 117-124.

Widdershoven, J.A.M. (1987) Vitamin K deficiency in infancy, Thesis, Katholieke Universiteit Nijmegen, The Netherlands.

WHO - World Health Organisation (1989) WHO-co-ordinated interlaboratory quality control studies and analytical field studies, Regional office for Europe, FADL, Copenhagen.

# PARTICULATE AEROSOLS, INCINERATORS AND HEALTH

C.V. HOWARD
*University of Liverpool*
*Fetal & Infant Toxico-Pathology*
*P.O. Box 147*
*L69 7ZA Liverpool*
*UNITED KINGDOM*

## Summary

Even the most modern municipal waste incinerators (MWIs) emit an aerosol of ultrafine particles which current bag filter technology cannot abate. Collection efficiencies for particles < 2.5 μm are between 5 and 30 per cent. For particles of < 1 μm, collection efficiency, most particles will pass unabated. Ultrafine particles have been found to be chemically highly reactive, even when originating from a relatively unreactive bulk material. The massive surface area associated with a small mass of nanometre-sized particles can act as a catalytic surface for the secondary formation of organic compounds.

Recent research has shown that the inhalation of ultrafine particles is associated with changes in the coagulability of the blood and this has been connected with epidemiological findings of increased cardiovascular disease in populations exposed to higher than average $PM_{10}$ exposure. The relative toxicity of ultrafine particles arising from different processes remains unresearched. However, metal nanoparticles have been shown to be particularly chemically reactive and it can be argued that MWIs, which have a heterogeneous input, high in heavy metals and halogenated organic materials, will tend to produce a more toxic ultrafine particulate aerosol than, say, a coal fired power station.



*P. Nicolopoulou-Stamati et al. (eds.), Health Impacts of Waste Management Policies,* 155–174.

There is an urgent requirement for research into the environmental and health impacts of the particulate aerosols emitted by current incinerators, which, because of the large volumes of gas they produce, have a significant local effect on air quality. Severe restrictions on the emissions of particulate aerosols, in the light of current health data, should become an integral part of future authorisations for the operation of MWIs.

## 1. Introduction

The process of incineration starts with a mass of matter, for the purposes of this discussion municipal waste, and transforms it into gases, particles and ash. The mass at the beginning and end of this process is identical. An indicative mass balance for a modern incinerator is included in Figure 23. However, a decrease in volume of the original waste is achieved through dispersion of gases and particulate aerosols to the environment. The levels of decrease in waste volume are broadly equivalent to those that would be achieved by simply separating and drying the compostables together with the high levels of compaction of the other wastes that are possible with modern steel wheeled compactors. The gases, particles and ash tend to be toxic, the level of toxicity depending upon the nature of the inputs and the operating conditions within the incinerator.

In 1996, most municipal waste incinerators (MWIs) in the EU had to be closed down and/or redesigned and retrofitted with improved gas cleaning equipment, to meet with new emission criteria required by Directive 89/429/EEC on the reduction of air pollution from existing municipal waste incineration plants. The Directive required that existing incinerators with a capacity of more than 6 tons per hour should be brought up to the 'new plant' standards required by Directive 89/369/EEC. For dust, this mandated an upper allowable emission level of 30 $mg/m^3$. This massive change and associated expenditure was necessary largely because of the acceptance, following years of debate, that MWIs had historically caused up to 80 per cent of dioxin contamination in parts of Europe. The main problems that have been identified to date in association with incineration are the dispersion of heavy metals (e.g. mercury, cadmium, lead) and persistent organic pollutants (POPs - e.g. dioxins, PCBs). Redesign of MWIs, with high temperature combustion chambers, rapid temperature quenching of the effluent gas stream, activated carbon injection and aqueous lime sparging have managed to reduce, but not eliminate, these pollutants from the stack emissions of MWIs.

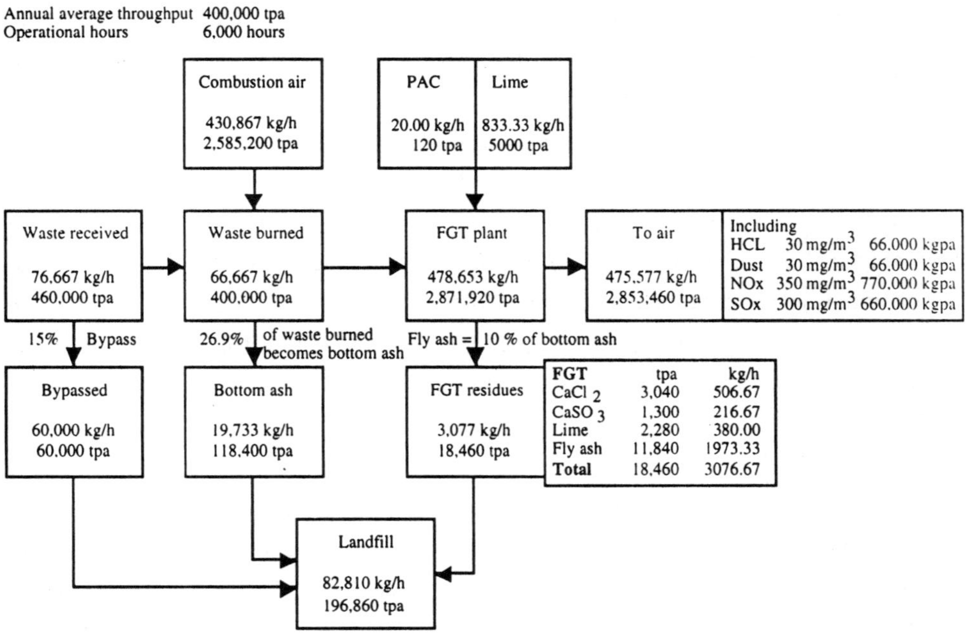


*Figure 23.* Mass balance of a modern incinerator, based on current technical specifications (after Watson, 1997)

The contribution of the particulate aerosols in the dispersion of these pollutants remains an understudied subject area. While the introduction of dioxins to the environment has been recognised as a global problem, through the mechanism of long-range transport, particulate aerosols pose a more local pollution burden. There are indications that some of the modern abatement equipment - particularly ammonia injection in an attempt to reduce emissions of oxides of nitrogen - may increase the emissions of the finest and most dangerous particulate aerosols (11th report HL Paper 71, 15th June 1999).

## 2. Properties of Respirable Particulate Aerosols

Animal and plant life as we know it evolved in the presence of particulate matter. Naturally occurring particles of less than 10 μm ($PM_{10}$) do occur, mainly in the form of resuspended sea salts. These pose no health threat and, if inhaled, are simply absorbed into the body. However, the size distribution of the majority of other naturally occurring particles, produced primarily by windborne soil erosion products and plant pollens, are quite large, certainly larger than those particulates of < 20 μm which are considered 'respirable'. The muco-ciliary carpet lining the airways has evolved to cope with an environmental loading of such naturally produced aerial particles. When humans started to use fire domestically, exposure to smaller particles, $PM_{10}$ and less, must have occurred on a regular basis. The retention and clearance of particles in the lung has been measured by stereological methods (Howard and Reed, 1998) in experimental animals by Geisser *et al.* (1990).

The advent of industrialised society has seen a vast increase in the level of combustion around the world, to the extent that it is now affecting the global level of carbon dioxide. This adds to the environmental $PM_{10}$ burden by the addition of primary and secondary particles which, with marine aerosol accounts for most of this class of particles. These three sources each contribute about 1/3$^{rd}$ of the total $PM_{10}$ burden in the UK (Deacon *et al.*, 1997; Harrison *et al.*, 1997). While recognising that there would have been naturally- and man-made combustion processes in the pre-industrial age, the level of particulate production would have been very small by comparison with today.

The size of the particulates produced by a process is closely tied to their ability to cause damage to the lung and other systems in the body as indicated in Table 14.

Nanoparticles are very small pieces of matter defined as having dimensions less than $10^{-8}$ m. They constitute a small proportion of the mass of almost all types of particulate material. They also constitute the majority of the number of particles found in aerosols produced as a result of combustion processes. Their importance in the field of catalyst manufacturing, where their high surface area has a very great influence on reactivity, is widely known (Jefferson and Tilley, 1999). However, at present we know relatively little about their detailed structure, or their chemical and physical properties.

*Table 14.* An indication of particle size and associated pathology.

| Source | Size distribution | Effect |
|---|---|---|
| Natural | > 20 μm | Minimal, some allergies, little systemic absorption |
| μ-milling | 1 - 10 μm | Occupational 'dust' diseases, some absorption systemically |
| Combustion | 1 nm - 10 μm | Major systemic absorption via lungs. Measurable health effects in the general population |

It is only in the last twenty years, with the advent of high-resolution electron microscopy (HREM) at sub-0.2 nm levels, and the consequent ability to resolve inter-atomic spacings at this level, that any real attempt has been made to determine the atomic structure of ***individual*** particles. What has been learned is that these minute particles have an increasing proportion of surface atoms as the particle size decreases. This leads to imbalances between the number of atoms and number of electrons present and hence the particles can be electrically charged. Thus they tend to have a higher chemical reactivity. In addition, novel configurations of atoms have been demonstrated in nanoparticles, which cannot exist in the bulk material (Jefferson and Tilley, 1999).

Although the ultrafine fraction of a particulate mixture will usually represent only a small proportion of the mass of the particles present, when the total surface area of the particles in an aerosol are considered, a very high proportion will consist of the highly chemically reactive surface of the smallest ultrafine particles. It is on this surface that catalytic reactions, such as the formation of halogenated organic molecules, can occur. Some of the most reactive nanoparticles to have been studied to date are metals (Jefferson and Tilley, 1999).

## 3. Health Effects of Ultrafine Particulate Aerosols

The effect of mixtures of particles of differing chemical composition entering the blood stream via the lungs in large numbers on a daily basis is only just beginning to be investigated. There is no doubt that some particulate aerosols are indeed hazardous. For example the mutagenic and carcinogenic nature of the constituents of some particles is recognised, PAHs being able to absorb onto the surface of fine particles (see Table 40 in the concluding chapter). However, the degree of hazard associated with specific types of particle and the precise mechanisms by which exposure leads to pathology are as yet poorly understood and are currently the subject of increasingly intense research.

According to researchers at Harvard University's School of Public Health, (Dockery and Pope, 1994) air pollution from combustion processes in cars, lorries and power plants, is killing roughly 60,000 Americans each year. This represents about 3 per cent of all U.S. deaths every year. Every combustion source is contributing to the death toll; none is benign, including:

- incinerators;
- soil burners;
- flares and after-burners;
- industrial and residential heaters and boilers;
- cars;
- buses;
- trucks;
- power plants.

The culprit appears to be the ultra fine particles created by combustion. Fine particles are not captured efficiently by modern pollution-control equipment. Furthermore, they are not visible except as a general haze. According to more than a dozen studies, there seems to be no threshold, i.e. no level of fine-particle pollution below which no deaths occur. The Harvard researchers have found that even air pollution levels that are well within legal limits are causing mortality and morbidity, especially among older people and those with chronic heart and lung ailments. In addition, studies indicate that fine-particle pollution is causing or exacerbating a wide range of human health problems, including:

- initiating and worsening asthma, especially in children;
- increasing hospital admissions for bronchitis, asthma and other respiratory diseases;
- increasing emergency room visits for respiratory diseases;
- reducing lung function (though modestly) in healthy people as well as (more seriously) in those with chronic diseases;

- increasing upper respiratory symptoms (runny or stuffy nose; sinusitis; sore throat; wet cough; head colds; hay fever; and burning or red eyes);
- increasing lower respiratory symptoms (wheezing; dry cough; phlegm; shortness of breath; and chest discomfort or pain);
- heart disease (Dockery and Pope, 1994).

Since 1987, the US Environmental Protection Agency (EPA) has been measuring $PM_{10}$ air pollution. The size of the particles is the most important issue from a public health viewpoint.

- Particles larger than 10 μm generally get caught in the nose and throat, never entering the lungs.
- Particles smaller than 10 μm can get into the large upper branches just below the throat where they are caught and removed (by coughing and spitting or by swallowing).
- Particles smaller than 5 μm can get into the bronchial tubes, at the top of the lungs.
- Particles smaller than 2.5 μm in diameter can get down to the deepest (alveolar) portions of the lungs where gas exchange occurs between the air and your blood stream, oxygen moving in and carbon dioxide moving out (Dockery and Pope, 1994; Seaton *et al.*, 1995).

These latter are potentially the most dangerous particles, because the deepest (alveolar) portions of the lung have no efficient mechanisms for removing them. If these particles are soluble in water, they pass directly into the blood stream within minutes. If they are not soluble in water, they are collected by scavenging cells called macrophages and then transported to lymph nodes where they are retained in the deep lung for long periods (months or years) (NRC, 1979). About 60 per cent of $PM_{10}$ particles (by weight) have a diameter of 2.5 μm or less (Dockery and Pope, 1994) whilst the 'vast majority' of the particles emitted from most waste incinerators will be of this size or smaller. These are the particles that can enter the human lung directly. (They also enter homes; indoor air and outdoor air typically contain the same quantities of fine particles, so buildings provide no refuge.)

In a modern city or major town, on many days, the air will contain 100 billion ($10^{11}$) one-nanometer-diameter particles in each cubic meter of air, all of them invisible (Seaton *et al.*, 1995). By weight, these 100 billion particles will only amount to 0.00005 micrograms (one ten-thousandth of 1 percent of the 50-microgram legal limit), yet they may be responsible for much of the health damage created by fine-particle pollution.

For this reason, in 1979, the National Research Council (US) said that measuring particles by weight, without regard to particle size, has 'little utility for judging effects'. (NRC, 1979). Particle size is a vital consideration when it comes to air pollution and health. The study of fine particles and their effects on human health has been under way in earnest since 1975. During the past 20 years, studies have been able to rule out sulphur dioxide and ozone pollution as the cause of the observed deaths (Dockery and Pope, 1994).

A study of 552,138 adult Americans in 151 metropolitan areas confirmed once again that there is a clear relationship between fine-particle air pollution and human deaths, and it ruled out smoking as a cause of the observed deaths (Pope *et al.*, 1995). This study is particularly important because it didn't simply match death certificates with pollution levels; It actually examined the characteristics (race, gender, weight and height) and lifestyle habits of all 552,138 people. Thus the study was able to rule out tobacco smoking (cigarettes, pipe and cigar); exposure to passive smoke; occupational exposure to fine particles; body mass index (relating to a person's weight and height); and alcohol use.

This study also controlled for changes in outdoor temperature. It found that fine-particle pollution was related to a 15 per cent to 17 per cent difference in death rates between the least polluted cities and the most-polluted cities. Researchers have shown previously that fine particles cause death and disease, but the mechanism by which this occurs has remained a mystery. A new hypothesis, published in the medical journal the Lancet (Seaton *et al.*, 1995) suggests that the particles retained in the deep lung cause inflammation which, in turn, releases natural chemicals into the blood stream causing coagulation of the blood. This hypothesis was proposed as a biological mechanism by which fine particles cause respiratory and heart-related diseases and death. It has recently received supporting evidence from the work of Donaldson *et al.* (1999), who have demonstrated a persistent rise in blood coagulability in rats following a single exposure to an aerosol of $PM_{10}$ particles. The precise mechanism remains elusive but it appears that the classical toxicological approach of determining a dose-response curve is not appropriate. The data indicates that there is probably a low exposure threshold, above which the effects described above will occur. The fact that the main end point under investigation, with respect to environmental particulate exposure, is arterial damage is consistent with the known fact that smokers, who voluntarily inhale particulate aerosols, almost all sustain arterial damage themselves (Auerbach, 1965).

A US EPA report (1996) addressing air quality for particulate matter reported that '*the PM studies do show effects related to exposure to the fine $PM_{2.5}$fraction, but high correlations among $PM_{2.5}$, $PM_{10}$, and acid aerosols make it very difficult to attribute the effects to a single specific exposure indicator*'. This highlights problems associated with trying to assess the effects of complex mixtures of particles from a variety of sources, through the use of the relatively blunt tool of human epidemiological studies. However the report goes on to say; '*Additional consideration of the subdivision of PM into fine and coarse components is also warranted. Indices of exposure that have been most consistently associated with health endpoints are by $PM_{10}$ or $PM_{2.5}$ and fine particle indicators. Less consistent relationships have been observed for total suspended particulate (TSP) and the coarse fractions of $PM_{2.5\text{-}10}$*'.

## 4. Incinerators and Particulate Aerosol Emissions

The most recent generation of MWIs (post 1996) have very expensive and sophisticated gas cleaning equipment. Environmental and human health protection from the adverse health effects associated with MSW effluvia depend entirely upon the bag filters and wet and dry scrubbing devices working to specification all the time. The experience with MWIs, however, does not give much confidence. For example, all of the UK plants that are currently operating under IPC authorisation, including the flagship 400,000 tpa SELCHP in South East London (see 'Incinerator emissions breaches focus attention on PVC' ENDS 292, May 1999 p. 13), regularly exceed the limits authorised by the Environment Agency – and without any sanction. Self reported figures from municipal waste incinerator operators show 499 breaches of emission limits between January 1996 and Autumn 1998, an average of more than 50 failures per plant (See House of Commons Written Answers, 9/11/1998 cols. 6-8, ENDS 286, November 1998 p. 30).

The Royal Bournemouth Hospital clinical waste incinerator was commissioned in March 1996 and appeared to work to specification initially. However, on monitoring hydrogen chloride vapour emission levels some seven months later, the concentration of HCl in the gases was found to be nearly five times the permitted level and this could have been going on for weeks. In Belgium, the technically upgraded MWI of Ostend, a textbook example of BAT, emitted up to 100 times the legal amount of dioxins of 0.1 ng/Nm$^3$ for more than three months after its inauguration in December 1997. This is the reality of operating MSW plants. The nature of the operating conditions, involving hot highly corrosive acid gases, means that malfunctions are to be expected.

Under the assumption that an MWI with all the latest equipment, including bag house filters, SNRC, activated carbon injection, etc., is working fully to specification - what is happening with respect to the particulate aerosol being emitted? The data in Table 15 was presented in support of an application to operate a new incinerator in the UK.

*Table 15.* Efficiency of bag house filters for particles of differing sizes as claimed by operators. (IPC Application, 1999).

| Particle size | Collection efficiency |
|---|---|
| $PM_{10}$'s | between 95% and 98% |
| $PM_{2.5}$'s | between 65% and 70% |
| PM below 2.5 | between 5% and 30% |

It is clear that the collection efficiency of current gas cleaning technologies falls sharply as particle size drops below a mean aerodynamic diameter of 2.5 μm. For particles of less than 1 μm, there will be a very low capture efficiency and for particle size below 0.2 μm, the abatement efficiency will be close to zero. Thus these plants, which have very high gas fluxes, are guaranteed to produce a chemically reactive ultrafine particulate aerosol.

An indication of the toxicity of dusts produced by municipal waste incineration is demonstrated in a paper which shows that workers may be exposed to mutagenic compounds from gaseous and particulate emissions and during ash removal operations

(Scarlett *et al.*, 1990). The frequency of urinary mutagens was measured by the Ames test among a sample of 104 refuse incinerator workers in seven incinerator plants during March-May 1988. Incinerator workers had a significantly higher risk for urinary mutagens and promutagens, as compared to water plant workers, after controlling for age. Among incinerator workers, increased risk of having urinary mutagens was associated with workers who wore protective clothing (defined as clothing other than masks or gloves) or whose job classification was equipment repair. It also showed a weak positive association with increasing age. There was an increased risk of urinary promutagens associated with not wearing gloves. The presence or absence of mutagenicity in workers' urine varied with plant location. Incinerator operating conditions affecting the production of toxicants and mutagens are discussed and the results of other studies involving toxicant exposure of humans near incinerators are cited.

There is little known about the relative toxicities of particulate aerosols from different processes.

## 5. Setting Municipal Waste Particulate Aerosol Emissions in Context with Vehicle Emissions

Burning municipal waste produces c. 5,140 Nm$^3$ per ton (HMIP, 1995) of emission gases. The emission limit for particulates in incinerator gases is 30 mg/Nm$^3$. The particulate emission per ton of waste incinerated, in grams, is therefore up to:

$$5{,}140 \text{ Nm}^3/\text{te} \times (30\text{mg/Nm}^3 / 1{,}000)$$
$$= 154.2 \text{ g/te of particulates.}$$

The EC Stage II indirect diesel particulate emission standard (Royal Commission on Environmental Pollution, 1994) is 0.08 g per kilometre travelled. The equivalent number of kilometres travelled for burning one ton of municipal waste is therefore:

$$154.2 \text{ g/te} / 0.08\text{g/km}$$
$$= 1{,}927.5 \text{ km/te}$$

Thus for a 400,000 tpa incinerator, such as SELCHP, the aggregate impact is equivalent 1,927.5 x 400,000 = 771 million vehicle kilometres per year. This type of consideration may well be of importance to decision-makers in moderating policy with respect to MWI plants.

A recently reported incinerator exceedance for particulates from the new NEM Teeside plant (UK Environment Agency IPC public register data) showed the daily average particulate emission level from Stack 1 for the 24 hour period ending 08.00 hrs 16 March 1999 was recorded as 55 $mg/m^3$. This is equivalent to an additional 28.8 kg particulates above the maximum level, based on a flow rate of 75,000 $m^3/h$. As can be seen above, that equates to the emissions from a diesel car driving 360,000 km. Thus relatively small or short-lived perturbations in performance, which are known historically to be common, can give rise to serious environmental impacts.

## 6. Putting a Price on the Costs of Incineration

Government agencies have been slow to admit that there are any possible health or cost disbenefits associated with municipal waste incineration. However there have recently been indications that regulators do rely on calculations associating these technologies with the number of deaths they are likely to cause and the degree of morbidity that might be expected in the local population.

In the UK, the Department of the Environment, Transport and the Regions (DETR) has released the final version of its 'Regulatory and Environmental Impact Assessment of the Proposed Waste Incineration Directive' or REIA (Ritchie *et al.*, 1999). This document clearly indicates that, in spite of the claims to the contrary, 'new' incinerators are not 'safe'. Even if the existing plants had been in compliance with their authorisations, (as assumed in the REIA) then alignment of the 1996 standards with those in the Hazardous Waste Incineration Directive would result each year in the deferment of 60 deaths in the UK and the avoidance or deferment of some 110 respiratory hospitalisations.

The corollary of this REIA is that over the past five years there have been of the order of 300 deaths and 550 respiratory hospitalisations that are calculated to have been caused by 'safe' incinerators. If this level of impact had been attributed, for example, to a fault in a consumer product then it would, quite rightly, have been forced off the market and probably be subject to massive liability claims.

When the public has already been misled on the possible risks from modern incinerators, it is not surprising that there is scepticism that the latest 'new' incinerators are - finally - really 'safe'. Operation of plant at tighter emission standards is effectively plotting a dose-response curve in a badly controlled experiment.

The REIA indicates, inter alia, that the human health benefits of the proposed directive (taking into account only acute effects) are as described in Table 16.

*Table 16.* Human health benefits associated with emission reductions due to the proposed incineration directive (after Ritchie *et al.*, 1999).

| **Pollutant** | **Numbers of deaths not brought forward** | **Number of respiratory hospital admissions avoided or not brought forward** | **Reduction in emissions on which these are based (tons)** | **N° of deaths not brought forward per ton of abated emissions** | **N° of respiratory hospital admissions avoided or not brought forward** |
|---|---|---|---|---|---|
| Ozone (from $No_x$) | 46 pa | 91 pa | 2264 | 0.02/t | 0.04/t |
| $SO_2$ | 5 pa | 6 pa | 1024 | 0.005/t | 0.006/t |
| Particulates | 0.2-0.3 pa | 0.4-0.5 pa | 141 | 0.002/t | 0.003/t |
| **Total** | **51 pa** | **97 pa** | | | |

Table 16 looks only at those deaths or hospital admissions (per year) avoided by the proposed improvement in standards of emissions to those in the proposed Directive.

The REIA does not examine how many deaths would still be brought forward by the operation of incinerators at the proposed Directive standard or by new incinerators that may come on line. To calculate these data is a fairly straightforward exercise based on the information provided in the REIA.

In the context of, for example, a 400,000 tpa incinerator, Table 16 could be adapted with the assumption that the authorised emission standards were being met. The results of these adaptation are provided in Table 17.

*Table 17.* Estimated human health costs of the introduction of a 400,000 tpa incinerator which is assumed to meet the proposed emissions standards (after Ritchie *et al.*, 1999).

| **Pollutant** | **Increase in emissions (tons pa)** | **N° of deaths brought forward** | **N° of respiratory hospital admissions brought forward** | **Number of deaths brought forward** | **Number of respiratory hospital admissions, new or brought forward** |
|---|---|---|---|---|---|
| Ozone (from $No_x$) | 440 | 0.02/t | 0.04/t | 8.8 pa | 17.6 pa |
| $SO_2$ | 220 | 0.005/t | 0.006/t | 1.1 pa | 1.32 pa |
| Particulates | 15.5 | 0.002/t | 0.003/t | 0.03 pa | 0.05 pa |
| **Total** | | | | **9.93 pa** | **18.87 pa** |

There is an uncertainty band on this data and the confidence envelope that can be attached to the results are detailed on pages 6 and 7 of the REIA Report which concludes that:

> *'Therefore there is greater uncertainty attached to the estimates of health and environmental benefits compared with the cost estimates. With so many contributing factors it is difficult to predict the level of uncertainty. A very conservative estimate would be ± one order of magnitude though we would expect the range to be narrower'.*

Consequently, the range of number of deaths brought forward by a single 400,000 tpa incinerator could range from 0.99 to 99 per year and the number of respiratory hospital admissions caused or brought forward could be 1.9 to 190 per year. Extended over a 25-year operational lifetime, the range of deaths extrapolates to between 25 and 2,475. Respiratory hospital admissions would range between 47 and 4,750 over the life of such an incinerator, given the DETR figures.

The REIA further emphasises that:

> *'It is stressed that the benefit estimates in this report are those that can be quantified with a reasonable degree of certainty. These will be underestimates of the total benefits as several other benefits (see section 4.2) have not been quantified.'*

These unquantified impacts explicitly exclude the impacts of chronic health effects due to dioxins and certain heavy metals, as well as excluding other morbidity effects apart from the limited respiratory effects. On the environmental front they exclude reductions in ecosystem damage due to acidification, in the risk of surface water, groundwater and soil contamination, and in environmental risks generally. In the context of potential new emissions the full disbenefits will therefore have been underestimated by simply using the data in the REIA.

The assessment undertaken for the European Commission on the draft Directive (AEA, 1997) is not so explicit in terms of numbers of deaths, but it does help to give a relative scale by attempting to quantify the impacts. For the very limited emissions that are considered and costed (there is too little data for many of the chemical compounds), then the damages are in the range of 10-60 ECU per ton of waste incinerated. Incorporation of the chronic effects of primary and secondary particles raises this to a range of 30-180 ECU per ton of waste incinerated.

Total health damages due to chronic effects of primary and secondary particles alone from a single 400,000 ton/year incinerator is therefore estimated to cost up to 48,000,000 ECU/year. Over a 25-year operational life, this results in up to a 1.2 billion ECU health disbenefit just from particulates. Even at the lowest range, the externality would be 8,000,000 ECU/year from particulates alone, 12,000,000 ECU/year for the total emissions for which impacts were assessed.

## 7. Conclusions

One might ask why steps weren't taken long ago to prevent the disease and death associated with fine-particle pollution, by specifying emission standards that related to particle size. After all, the National Academy of Sciences said as early as 1979 that '... *alveolar retention of relatively insoluble particles is recognised to be important to the pathogenesis of chronic lung disease* ...' (NRC, 1979). In other words, the Academy was convinced many years ago that fine particles retained in the deep lung cause long-term lung disease. The Academy said at that time, '*In summary, particulate atmospheric pollutants may be involved in chronic lung disease pathogenesis as causal factors in chronic bronchitis, as predisposing factors to acute bacterial and viral bronchitis, especially in children and cigarette smokers, and as aggravating factors for acute bronchial asthma and the terminal stages of oxygen deficiency (hypoxia) associated with chronic bronchitis and/or emphysema and its characteristic form of heart failure (cor pulmonale)*'. (NRC, 1979). If the Harvard researchers are correct in their estimate, that 60,000 Americans die each year from fine-particle pollution, and tens of thousands more are made sick (especially children), then we can calculate that, since 1979, nearly a million Americans (960,000) have been killed by fine particle pollution, and millions more have suffered morbidity.

This is consistent with the evidence given by the UK Environment Minister, Michael Meacher, to the House of Lords that:

> '*Q440 ... I repeat that the emissions from incinerator processes are extremely toxic. Some of the emissions are carcinogenic. We know scientifically that there is no safe threshold below which one can allow such emissions.*'

This statement from the Minister should signal the need for great caution in assessing the locations and the potential impacts for any waste management facilities which could include an element of incineration.

The Lords concluded their report by commenting that:

> *'114. We are concerned that the links between pollution control and public health are not being systematically addressed; there is a lack of clarity over where the primary responsibility lies. The Environment Agency, SEPA and EHS (DOENI) admit that they depend on external expertise to perform their required functions in assessing the potential impacts of waste incineration on human health. Bearing in mind the agencies' responsibilities under part 1 of the Environmental Protection Act 1990 and related legislation we find this disquieting ... we were not convinced that there was an effective flow of information at the "sharp end".'*

Politely indicating that the Environment Agency have probably not been 'discharging their functions' with the Relevant Objectives of protecting health, the Lords go on, not surprisingly in view of this conclusion, to give support to the public concerns about emissions including dioxins and particulates from new incinerators:

> *'110 ... when the precautionary principle is applied, we think that it would be wrong to discount public concern about the health implications of incineration products (especially dioxins) on the grounds that it is derived from the experience of an older generation of municipal incinerators which the 1989 Directives have essentially done away with. Although considerable progress has been made in understanding the toxicology and exposure effects of many of the key pollutants, continued epidemiological work will be needed. We consider there are well established grounds for caution, justifying the general approach of the draft Directive. We feel that the collection and study of data on the potential health risks from combustion products should continue to be a priority. In particular in the light of the evidence from health professionals about emissions of particles of ammonium nitrate below $PM_{2.5}$, and their behaviour in the body, ...'*

The secondary particulates, including ammonium nitrate particles, are calculated to be the greatest source of damage. They arise, at least in part, however, from the air pollution control devices of incinerators, including the injection of urea to reduce emissions of oxides of nitrogen.

In a society which depends heavily upon combustion processes for power production, transport and heavy industry, a world without anthropogenic particulate aerosols is unrealistic and unobtainable in the foreseeable future. Further objective multidisciplinary research will aid decision-makers in their task of optimising cost and benefit. It may in future be proved to be that some processes contribute a disproportionate amount of the toxic burden attributable to the $PM_{10}$ fraction. For example, municipal waste incinerators, which have appreciable heavy and transitional metal contents in their feedstocks, are likely to be more damaging than coal fired power stations, for each unit of energy produced. And yet there does not appear to have been any systematic analysis of respective $PM_{10}$ effluvia of different industries with respect to the basic physical chemistry or the types of health effects that have been discussed in this book. This become should become an urgent aim for research.

## Acknowledgement

The author wishes to acknowledge the input of Alan Watson, of Public Interest Consultants, for his helpful comments and additions on a number of aspects of this paper.

## References

AEA (1997) *Economic Evaluation of the Draft Incineration Directive, December 1996*, European Commission, ISBN 92-828-0083-0.

Auerbach, O., Cuyler Hammond, E., and Garfinkel, L. (1965) Smoking in relation to artherosclerosis of the coronary arteries, *New England Journal of Medicine* **273**, 775-779.

Deacon, A.R., Derwent, R.G., Harrison, R.M., Middleton, D.R., and Moorcroft, S. (1997) Analysis and interpretation of measurements of suspended particulate matter at urban background sites in the United Kingdom, *Sci. Total Environ.* **203**, 17-36.

Dockery, D.W., and Pope, C.A. III (1994) Acute respiratory effects of particulate air pollution, *Annual Review of Public Health* **15**, 107-132.

Donaldson, J., Stone, V., and MacNee, W. (1999) The toxicology of ultrafine particles, in R.L. Maynard and C.V. Howard (eds) *Particulate Matter: Properties and Effects Upon Health*, BIOS Scientific Publishers Ltd., Oxford, UK, pp. 115-129, ISBN 1-85996-172X.

Geiser, M., Cuz Orive, L.M., Hof, V.I., and Gehr, P. (1990) Assessment of particle retention and clearance in intrapulmonary conducting airways of hamster lungs with the fractionator, *J. Microscopy* **160**, 75-88.

HMIP (1995), Risk assessment of dioxin releases from municipal waste incineration processes, section 7.6.3., HMSO, London.

Harrison, R.M., Deacon, A.R., and Jones, M.R. (1997) Sources and processes affecting concentrations of $PM_{10}$ and $PM_{2.5}$ particulate matter in Birmingham, UK, *Atmos. Eviron.* **32**, 4103-4117.

Howard, C.V., and Reed, M.G. (1998) *Unbiased Stereology, Three-dimensional Measurement in Microscopy*, BIOS Scientific Publishers, Oxford.

IPC Application (1999) by Onyx Hampshire to operate a municipal waste incinerator at Portsmounth, September 1999, supplementary information, p. 20. Efficiency of bag house filters for particles of differing sizes, as claimed by operators.

Jefferson, D.A., and Tilley, E.E.M. (1999) The structural and physical chemistry of nanoparticles, in R.L. Maynard and C.V. Howard (eds) *Particulate Matter: Properties and Effects Upon Health*, BIOS Scientific Publishers Ltd., Oxford, UK, pp. 63-84, ISBN 1-85996-172X.

NRC - National Research Council, National Academy of Sciences (1979) *Airborne Particles*, University Park Press, Baltimore, Md., pp. 108-110.

Pope, C.A. III, Thun, M.J., Namboodiri, M.M., Dockery, D.W., Evans, J.S., Speizer, F.E., and Heath, C.W. Jr. (1995) Particulate air pollution as a predictor of mortality in a prospective study of US adults, *American Journal of Respiratory and Critical Care Medicine* **151**, 669-674.

Ritchie, A.N. *et al.* (1999) Regulatory and environmental impact assessment of the proposed Waste Incineration Directive - final report, ENTEC UK for UK Department of the Environment, Transport and the Regions, DETR report n° 99019.

Royal Commission on Environmental Pollution (1994) 18th Report, Transport Cm2674, HMSO, London, October 1994.

Seaton, A., MacNee, W., Donaldson, K., and Godden, D. (1995) Particulate air pollution and acute health effects, *The Lancet* **345**, 176-178.

US EPA (1996) Air Quality Criteria for Particulate Matter, EPA/600/P-95/001aF, bF and cF (three volumes).

Watson, A. (1997) Personal communication.

# HEALTH AND ENVIRONMENTAL IMPACT ASSESSMENT

L. HENS
*Vrije Universiteit Brussel*
*Human Ecology Department*
*Laarbeeklaan 103*
*B-1090 Brussel*
*Belgium*

## Summary

Waste deposit sites and incinerators, the two main disposal routes of waste today, raise important health concerns. Therefore, the questions if and to what extent new projects in the waste management area will result in potential health damage are most relevant.

This paper describes how to deal with these questions. Two main aspects are considered:

a. the health impact assessment (HIA) methodology, which allows the forecasting of possible health effects of new projects, plans, programmes or policies;
b. the integration of HIA into the general environmental impact assessment process. In particular, the specific points on HIA to be addressed during the different procedural EIA steps are described.

HIA is analysed as a six-step process entailing the description of the project site in a way which allows the identification of the vulnerable groups to be studied; the identification of the changes in the environment relevant to the health of the population; the identification and quantification of the exposure and the dose; the prediction of the relevant health



*P. Nicolopoulou-Stamati et al. (eds.), Health Impacts of Waste Management Policies,* 175–197.

effects; the evaluation of these predictions; the mitigating measures and post project analysis including monitoring and surveillance.

Integrating HIA in EIA is a matter of focussing on the three main objectives of HIA (identification of health hazards, interpretation of these hazards as risks and management of the health risks) and their realisation throughout the EIA procedure. It is shown that in particular scoping, setting up the terms of reference, the preparation of the environmental impact statement, the public participation and the post project analysis are the main phases during which specific HIA elements need to be explicitly addressed.

Although the application of HIA looks like the most promising way to deal with important questions with which society confronts policy makers, its full application will strongly depend upon the application of good practice methods, more research, more attention to quality control in EIA and better targeted education and training on these subjects.

## 1. Introduction

Environmental impact assessment (EIA) for waste management policy options involves mainly waste deposit sites and incineration plants. In the future recycling centres might also become the subject of assessment studies. Strategic environmental assessment (SEA) in a waste management context aims at calculating the impacts of different policy scenarios and location alternatives. In both approaches, health is of critical concern. Waste deposit sites have been shown to be pollution blackspots world-wide. Uncontrolled or poorly-managed sites are associated with the generation of pests and the spreading of diseases. In controlled dumping sites, the leachate might contaminate the groundwater and the air in such a way that genetic aberrations (Hens, 1993) and congenital malformations (Dolk *et al.*, 1998) appear in the neighbouring populations. Incinerators spread, via the air and through ash, impressive amounts of pollutants which are either not destroyed by the incineration process (like heavy metals) or which are generated in the plant (like dioxins and furans) (Walker, 1991).

An overwhelming majority of EISs (Environmental Impact Statements) deal with these problems by calculating the expected emissions and stating that the existing standards will not be exceeded. This sounds like a convincing conclusion, allowing the project to go ahead. The legal character of standards also contributes to the appearance of reliability. However, such conclusions also obscure an important part of relevant considerations, such as, for example:

- For many substances and health-related situations (e.g. communicable diseases), no standards exist;
- Most (environmental) standards are based upon what is feasible in a best available technology (BAT) not entailing excessive costs (BATNEEC) framework, which has no direct health significance;
- Those standards based upon health considerations are not only based upon the results of toxicological and epidemiological studies, but also involve economic evaluation and social feasibility, which often dilute the health aspects;
- For carcinogenic substances, no 'safe' values exist and only a risk figure can be provided;
- No 'standard' person exists. People have different lifestyles, leading to different exposures, and different susceptibilities to particular hazards.

These are the main reasons why standards are difficult to handle and are an imperfect point of reference to evaluate health effects. Consequently, the failure to integrate, or even give attention to, the relationships between the biophysical environment and human health, remains a major deficiency in environmental impact statements world-wide. In the UK, a review examining coverage of impacts on human health in thirty-nine EISs estimated that potential health effects had received adequate coverage in approximately only 28 per cent of the statements studied. Although legislation requires environmental health issues to be addressed, this was clearly not seen as a priority by developers or consultants. The statements examined also failed to provide the information necessary to access the likely implications of new developments for health, and the populations at risk were rarely identified (BMA, 1998).

A similar, but more limited, study which evaluated the human health section in EISs in Flanders and the Netherlands, reached similar conclusions pointing to the current inadequate situation (Adang and De Stordeur, 1996).

To improve the integration of health issues in EIA, two elements are necessary:

a. an appropriate methodology to deal with (the most important) health risks in EIA or SEA. This methodology has been developed and is known as health impact assessment;
b. the implementation of this methodology in the environmental impact assessment process.

This contribution overviews both these aspects. The general objective is to improve both the effectiveness and the efficiency of EIA/SEA.

## 2. Health Impact Assessment (HIA) Methodology

### *2.1. Overview – A 6-Step Process*

Health risks can both increase and decrease as a result of a project, programme, plan or policy. A decrease in a health risk is one form of health benefit. Other health benefits might emerge when the project promotes health through mechanisms such as an improved standard of living. Most often, and in particular when it comes to the evaluation of waste management projects, however, HIA will have to address the potentially harmful impacts of the chemicals, biological and/or physical agents released by the new developments.

Integral to an understanding of this discussion is the distinction between a health hazard and a health risk. The following definitions apply:

a. A health hazard is anything that can cause harm (e.g. high voltage electricity electrocution: the harmful outcome is injury or death). Hazard assessment requires direct measurements;
b. A health risk is a measure of the likelihood that a health hazard will actually cause harm to a particular individual or group of people (e.g. the health risk of electricity depends on having a bare 'live' wire, a person ignorant or careless enough to touch it and the absence of warning signs. In view of the precautions, the risk is usually small). Risk assessment involves interpretation of hazard assessment data. Risk assessments are based upon assumption rather than on measurements. Their outcome can be qualitative or quantitative;

c. A health impact is any change in health risk that is reasonably attributable to a project, programme, plan or policy.

For a more in-depth discussion on hazards and risks, see Johnston *et al.* (1999) and Buekens *et al.* (1999).

The health risk assessment methodology can be summarised in six basic steps, which are represented in Table 18. These steps are described more in detail in the following sections.

*Table 18.* The six steps of HIA used in Flanders (after Janssens and Hens, 1995).

| | **EHIA in Flanders** |
|---|---|
| (1) | Description of the project site |
| (2) | Identification of changes in the environment relevant to the health of the population |
| (3) | Identification and qualification of the exposure and dose |
| (4) | Prediction of the relevant health effects |
| (5) | Evaluation of the predictions |
| (6) | Identification and evaluation of mitigating measures |

## *2.2. Description of the Project Site*

The description of the project site is an essential element of HIA. A visit to the site is indispensable to have a good, overall grasp of the lay of the project and its surroundings. The surroundings have many characteristics which can be important in the study of health effects due to environmental changes. The size of the area which needs to be studied depends on the features of the:

- project (substances and processes used, size of the project, geographical position, etc.);
- surroundings (topography, meteorological conditions, soil characteristics, history, etc.);

- inhabitants (demography, socio-economic status, land use, use of natural resources, health status, patterns of activity, individual differences, etc.).

Clearly, the report should not repeat elements described in previous sections, but rather build upon them. Only data relevant to understanding the health situation should be elaborated. Table 19 summarises the data which are considered fundamental in the description of the study area.

After an examination of these elements, it should be possible to identify groups at risk (potentially vulnerable groups). Such groups then merit special attention. This does not mean, of course, that other sub-populations should be ignored. As a rule, in particular children and elderly people are more vulnerable for the emissions of waste incinerators. Children and pregnant women are the traditional groups of increased risk in the analysis of waste deposit sites.

The content and scope of the EIA depend largely on the project description. This determines the size of the area to be studied and also the factors to be discussed. Often, a substance-oriented approach is the option which has been chosen. Marking the geographic area under investigation is an important step in EIA. In this way, the area will be confined physically, so that research can concentrate only on the land which is implicated. In order to do this, the experts need an extensive description of the project and of the surroundings (its landscape and inhabitants).

*Table 19.* Basic data describing the study area (Step 1).

| | |
|---|---|
| 1. | General description of the area: borders, social, geographical, economic aspects of the project, its importance for the (local) community |
| 2. | Physical conditions of the environment: climate, topography, soil, ... |
| 3. | History, description of existing pollution (sources) |
| 4. | Use of the area (agriculture, recreation, industry, residential, traffic situation, ...) and natural resources (ground and surface water, hunting, fishing, ...) |
| 5. | Demography: population density, age distribution, socio-economic composition, ethnic data, distribution of vulnerable groups |

### 2.3. *Identification of Changes in the Environment Relevant to the Health of the Population*

The project description must provide the experts with enough information to enable them to get a broad picture of the possible environmental changes which may occur as a result of implementing the project. Based on this description, it is possible to focus on how those changes can affect the health of the residents. Only relevant (significant) changes should be examined. These changes include not only substances (chemical factors) released into the environment but also physical factors (e.g. noise and vibration) and biological factors (e.g. micro-organisms, insects and other pests).

Table 20 provides a summarised overview of the relevant changes to be addressed. These changes should be described both in a qualitative and a quantitative way. As far as the latter issue is concerned, a comparison with the reference situation is essential. For HIA, the description of the reference situation depends on up-to-date morbidity and mortality data. For waste deposit sites, data on cancer and congenital malformations are minimal requirements. For incinerators, one also needs data on single/multiple pregnancies.

*Table 20.* Environmental effect groups, allowing for the identification of the relevant health status changes (step 2).

| | | |
|---|---|---|
| 1. | Noise emissions | Noise |
| 2. | Traffic | Traffic pressure<br>Safety |
| 3. | Air emissions, immissions, deposition | Air quality changes<br>Odour<br>Drinking water quality changes<br>Surface water quality changes<br>Soil quality changes |
| 4. | Water emissions | Drinking water quality changes<br>Surface water quality changes<br>Soil quality changes |
| 5. | Soil emissions | Drinking water quality changes<br>Soil quality changes |
| 6. | Acute accidents/calamities | Immediate physical danger |

Changes in human health should be interpreted in a general way. Not only do disease and discomfort need to be considered, but also changes in psychological and social well-being. It is, however, very difficult to quantify discomfort, nuisance or psychological effects.

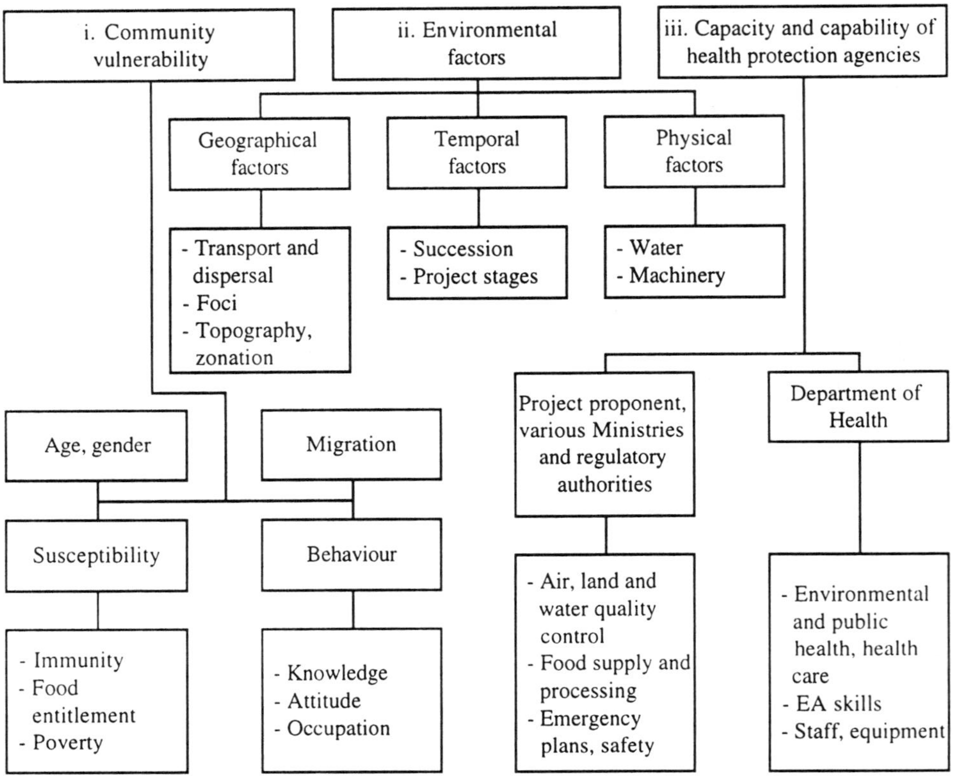


*Figure 24.* The main components of the assessment of change in health risk.

Currently there is some discussion on the scope of an EIA. While in most countries, EIAs (and consequently the associated HIAs) focus on effects resulting from changes in the physical environment, there exists a trend to broaden this scope to add social and institutional elements. In the literature, one finds references defining the more limited scope as environmental health impact assessment (EHIA). The broader, human ecology-targeted approach is described as characteristic for health impact assessment (HIA). In operational terms, the components for the assessment of health risks are:

1. community vulnerability: where communities are identified by those social components which are known to make them more or less vulnerable to disease. These components include age, gender, migration, susceptibility, and behaviour;
2. environmental factors: where those biophysical factors are identified that expose the vulnerable communities to health hazards. This part of the analysis corresponds to the narrower scope of an EIA explained above;
3. health protection agencies: where the capacity and capability of health protection agencies to safeguard the community is analysed.

A flowchart of this broader approach is represented in Figure 24.

### *2.4. Identification and Quantification of the Exposure Pathway and Dose*

Potential adverse health factors follow a specific pathway through the environment. This pathway starts from the production and emission of the compound. During passage through an environmental compartment (air, water, soil) the factor may undergo many changes (dilution, transformation, accumulation, etc.). Finally it will reach its target. Data of the exposure rely on estimations from the technical disciplines. The 'food basket' is equally important. For many pollutants, exposure through what we eat is more important than through what we drink, breathe or ingest through pica. In dioxin exposure cases, more than 90 per cent of the exposure is provided by food and less than 10 per cent by air, while the exposure through water is negligible. Table 21 summarises these data.

*Table 21.* Data allowing for the definition of the extent of exposure (step 3a).

1. Immission data which are the result of
   - emissions
   - transportation
   - transformation
   - elimination
2. Immission data in
   - air (including indoor air)
   - soil
   - drinking water
   - 'food basket'

The effect depends not only on the external concentration in the environment, but also on individual features. Physical exercise, feeding habits, age and gender are only some of these elements. When estimating the exposure, one has to take into account not only pollution released by the project but also the pollution which already exists because of other activities, past or present. Having a history of the project site helps experts to identify current or past sources and levels of pollution.

In the organism, the compound follows an analogous pathway: uptake (inhalation, ingestion or via the skin), transport, biotransformation, eventual accumulation and excretion. Somewhere along this pathway, it will eventually reach its target and exert the effect. Ideally, it should be possible to obtain a measurement of exposure at the level of the target (cell, tissue, organ). In most cases however, this is not feasible, so we have to use models and estimations.

### *2.5. Prediction of the Relevant Health Effects*

Prediction of the probability and seriousness of a health effect is the main aim of HIA. This is supported by toxicological and epidemiological research. The goal of this research is to establish a relationship between dose and effect.

Very often these dose-response data come from experiments on animals. Interpretation of the results necessitates extrapolation. This process is affected by uncertainty and requires safety factors. The relatively infrequent data on humans come from occupational and/or acute accidental exposure to high doses. HIA needs data from chronic, low-dose exposures, to make reliable predictions concerning the health impact of a project. More extrapolation is necessary when such data are not available, increasing the uncertainty of the predictions.

One of the difficulties which occurs in environmental toxicology is the assessment of the risk to human health posed by mixtures of chemicals. Health risks from mixtures can be the sum of the risks from the separate elements (addition). But substances can also interact in many ways. If this is the case, the risk from a cocktail of chemicals can be lower (antagonism) or higher (synergism) than the sum of the individual risks. A well-known example of synergism is the increase in the risk of contracting cancer owing to exposure to asbestos when the exposed individuals are also regular smokers. The evaluation of pollutants with a xenoestrogenic activity, which is relevant for both waste deposit sites and incinerators, is more difficult. Estimations of increases of cancer incidence and congenital malformations can be based upon epidemiological studies present in the literature. Both aspects are characterised, however, by important scientific uncertainty.

Epidemiological studies relate observations in existing populations to their environmental conditions. Care has to be taken to avoid being misled by spurious correlation. A numerical relation between two events does not mean explicitly that there is a causal link between the two events. Owing to the relative short time-span of an EIA only cross-sectional epidemiological studies are recommended.

The results of the toxicological and epidemiological studies can be summarised using the parameters listed below:

- name and code of the chemical substances (EU or any other code). This can be complemented by the chemical formula and additionally by current synonyms;
- acute toxicity ($LD_{50}$). Toxicity classification. Possible effects;
- subchronic toxicity. NOEL. Possible effects;
- chronic toxicity. NOEL. Possible effects;
- carcinogenicity (yes/no, IARC or EPA classification);
- mutagenicity (yes/no, test used);
- teratogenicity (yes/no, test used, NOEL);
- corrosiveness, irritation (classification);
- inflammability;
- explosiveness;
- available data concerning occupational risk (least dose that causes adverse health effects, doses without observed health effect, classification of the effects, etc.);
- available data concerning epidemiological studies and risks for the total population and specific subpopulations (see above);
- guidelines, standards (general population, occupational situations, environmental quality standards, other available standards);

- persistence in the environment (half-life in different environmental compartments, rate of breakdown, other persistence indices). Mostly orders of magnitude are sufficient;
- water/air-distribution coefficient;
- soil/water-distribution coefficient;
- degree of bio-accumulation (directly measured or estimated). If measured directly, the biological species should be mentioned. If estimated, the method should be mentioned;
- any other information that can be useful for this substance.

Zaponi (1989) suggested this list of data useful for HIA of chemical substances. During the study of most projects, several substances will be examined. The lists of all the relevant data can be combined in a matrix. This way, an overview can be created of the available information relevant for health risk analysis.

This list clarifies the available basic knowledge pollutant-by-pollutant. Most often, these data are also indicative of the lack of knowledge, in many cases. This completeness/lack of knowledge will determine whether the conclusion will be quantitative or qualitative. Quantitative answers are only possible if the quality of the numerical data is high and a model that combines the components is available. In the absence of such data and models, a more simple ranking of trends may be all that is practicable. This consists of a statement that a change in health risk is attributable to the project. It is recommended that the conclusion should be presented in several stages of increasing level of detail:

- A summary table, of which the outline is provided in Figure 25. The number of rows can be expanded to include all the health hazards;
- Summary justifications of the statements included in the table;
- More detailed presentation of the data and the assumptions on which the justifications are based.

### *2.6. Evaluation of the Predictions – Assessment of the Health Risks*

The results of the investigations described above need interpretation. Similar data might lead to very different outcomes for many reasons. Interpretation is also necessary because scientific data usually follow a statistical distribution. The evaluation by an expert should, in many cases, not be left out.

| Health hazard | Community group | Vulnerability of community group | Environmental factors determining exposure to the hazard | Capacity and capability of health protection agencies | Change in health risk attributable to the project |
|---|---|---|---|---|---|
| Communicable diseases | | | | | |
| Non-communi-cable diseases | | | | | |
| Injury | | | | | |
| Inappropriate nutrition | | | | | |
| Mental disorder | | | | | |

*Figure 25.* Model of summary health assessment table.

Effects on human health can be characterised in two different ways:

1. according to the nature of the effect: acute or chronic, reversible or irreversible, local or systemic, stochastic or non-stochastic;
2. according to the nature of the target: the nervous system, the liver, the kidneys, the respiratory tract, the reproductive system, etc.

Cancer should be given special attention. It is a typical stochastic effect. Although the extent of the effect is not dose-dependent, the probability of expression of the effect, on the other hand, is. As a rule, there is no threshold. Non-stochastic effects usually have a threshold. The intensity of the effect is dose-dependent.

HIA is based on the comparison of two sets of circumstances. The first one is the reference situation. In most cases, this will be a description of the current circumstances. The other wing of the comparison is the planned situation. This is a description of the environment when the project has been completed and is operational. To evaluate the health impact of a project, both the reference and the planned situation should be described in as detailed a manner as possible during the HIA process. With the current (reference) situation in mind, the expert tries to predict and evaluate the health effects owing to the planned changes. The predicted effects are grouped, in order to organise the discussion and evaluation better. During the evaluation process, one should get an idea of how extensive the effects in the planned situation are expected to be.

Every project has good and bad aspects which affect the health of the residents. HIA aims to weigh the pros and cons and to choose the alternative with a minimum burden on people's health. In waste management discussions, however, the pros have to do with the need for waste management and the general policy options. It is indeed a matter of general waste policy to determine what the contribution of incinerators, deposit sites, recycling, re-use and prevention will be. Therefore, a lot of prevention of disease depends upon the choices made at the political level. In optimising these choices, HIA in a context of SEA might be of significant help.

### 2.7. *Identification and Evaluation of Mitigating Measures – Health Risk Management*

Every activity has a certain impact on its environment. During EIA, several alternatives are evaluated and one will be selected. This selection is a compromise between possible impacts at different levels. The chosen alternative can result in some burden being placed on human health. HIA should be an integral part of EIA. This means that many other factors will also be examined, after the integration of all the different aspects and an evaluation of all the possible alternatives. This alternative is not necessarily the best from the point of view of the assessor concerned with health.

The primary goal of HIA is to avoid or else minimise any potential adverse effects on health from projects. The projects are studied before being initiated. This preventive approach allows the Government to take any appropriate actions in order to protect the environment and the health of the people that reside therein. Once the risks to health have been assessed, it is possible to recommend mitigating measures to minimise their impact. These measures should be evaluated on their feasibility. The principle of 'best available techniques not entailing excessive costs' (BATNEEC) should be applied.

Table 22 provides a list of the traditional operational instruments the HIA expert can act upon. Managing health risks is, however, more than the application of a set of instruments. For most projects, a health risk management strategy is required and the preparation of action plans to mitigate negative impacts (including health impacts) is a standard component of EIA. The objective of a health risk management plan is safeguarding health, mitigating health risks and seeking opportunities to improve health. It is a soundly thought-out mixture of well-selected instruments used at an appropriate time.

*Table 22.* Instruments for mitigating measures in HIA (step 5).

1. Limit emissions
    - changes in alternatives to production processes and/or import
    - water treatment, air treatment
    - give up project
2. Limit exposure
    - location alternatives
    - protection of residential areas (e.g. noise walls, zoning policy, ...)
    - protection from exposure (e.g. if water is main exposure source, provide alternatives to contaminated water exposure, ...)
    - inform population, with special attention for groups at risk
    - personal protection devices (e.g. iodine tablets for radioactive risks)
3. Medical infrastructure and emergencies
    - monitoring and early warning systems
    - disaster planning actions
    - emergency medicine facilities
4. Schemes to reimburse and redistribute losses
    - insurance

## 2.8. *Post-Project Monitoring, Post-Project Evaluation and Surveillance*

Post-monitoring means that the project is followed during its preparation, construction and implementation phases, and eventually during its demolition as well. The effects observed are compared to those predicted in the EIS. This evaluation offers an opportunity to refine the prediction methodology and allows the expert to obtain data for substances whose behaviour is not very well understood as yet. Especially when it comes to possible health effects of incinerators and waste deposit sites, the scientific uncertainty linked with the prediction of health effects is important. Prospective monitoring of key problems as cancer, congenital malformations, and multiple pregnancies might erode this problem.

Monitoring is however, not a legal requirement in most EU countries, but there is growing scientific consensus that it should be an integral part of EIA and SEA. Indeed, almost all projects with potentially adverse health effects require recommendation for post-project activities. Table 23 provides a list of the most often used instruments in this part of EIA. Monitoring and surveillance are the most commonly used.

*Table 23.* Instruments for post-project evaluation (step 6).

| | |
|---|---|
| 1. | Monitoring of chemical, physical, biological pollutants |
| 2. | Epidemiological surveillance |
| 3. | Registration of complaints |
| 4. | Advisory committee |
| 5. | Notification mechanisms, on occurence of malfunction |

Monitoring typically involves the measuring and recording of physical, biological, chemical, social and economic variables associated with the impacts which are expected (e.g. air, water and/or soil quality, noise, employment, revenue). It should not be limited to man, but might be extended to core issues in the food chain. For incinerators, which are expected to emit dioxins and furans, it is important to monitor their concentration in the milk of cows and sheep grazing in the vicinity of the plant.

Surveillance, on the other hand, aims at collecting information, e.g. on a specific health risk, that may contribute to future decisions and evaluations. It is of particular importance for vulnerable groups.

### *2.9. Scientific Uncertainty*

HIA however, faces many practical and theoretical problems. It depends for its primary data on other more technical disciplines. Predictions of effects on human health depend on scientific research. For many substances, such research is often scarce or has not been done. The data that do exist show variations which are typical of observations which follow statistical distributions. An HIA expert has also to take into account extensive individual variation in effects on health, due to personal habits and genetic variability. These sources of variation result in uncertainties which can not be neglected.

These scientific uncertainties and limitations should be made transparent in the report.

## 3. Incorporating HIA within EIA

### *3.1. Targets*

HIA necessitates not only a clear methodology. To be effective, the different steps need to be built explicitly into the EIA process. HIA should be made an integral component of EIA, not a separate or parallel activity.

HIA has basically a threefold purpose:

a. the identification of health hazards (and benefits) linked with the project;
b. the interpretation of health hazards as health risks which could be changed by the project;
c. contributing to the management of the health risks.

Action to reach each of these three targets needs to be initiated at different stages of the procedure.

### *3.2. Scoping*

The identification of the health hazards should always be part of the scope of an EIA. This inclusion should be systematic, specific and precise. This means that during the scoping process a detailed list is drawn up of the health hazards that should be investigated. There is currently no universal methodology for addressing the potential health effects of a project. As a starting point for the discussion, the British Medical Association (BMA, 1998) suggests grouping health hazards into five main categories. These categories are the following:

1. communicable disease, e.g. sexually transmitted diseases, infections, water-borne diseases, microbiological food contamination, etc.;
2. non-communicable disease, e.g. chronic poisoning, lung disease associated with dust or ozone, effects of noise, carcinogenic, mutagenic and teratogenic effects, etc.;
3. inappropriate nutrition, e.g. deprivation, access to food, pesticide or other chemical contamination, etc.;
4. injury, e.g. traffic injury, violence resulting from inner city decay, occupational injury;
5. mental disorders, e.g. stress, chronic depression and substance abuse.

### *3.3. Terms of Reference*

Once the health hazards associated with the project have been identified, the next step is to produce the terms of reference (ToR), which stipulate the required contents for the EIS. Making sure that health aspects are integrated into the EIA necessitates that the requirement to address health is explicitly addressed in the ToR. Moreover, these ToR should deal with the issue in sufficient detail, to avoid vague, general and unclear outputs on health. Sufficient detail here means basically two elements:

a. listing the potential health hazards identified during the scoping process;
b. mentioning the essentials of the six steps of the HIA procedure (Table 18).

It is a matter of good EIA practice that the results of the scoping phase and the terms of reference are open for public consultation and discussion.

This phase also concludes the realisation of the first objective: identification of health hazards (and benefits) associated with the project.

### 3.4. *Health in the EIS*

The second target to be accomplished, the interpretation of health hazards as health risks which could be changed by the project, is at the heart of the EIS. The problem can be handled by the six step EIA approach discussed in part 2 of this paper.

### 3.5. *Public Participation*

Public debates about risk are difficult for many reasons. It is now widely accepted that the best option is full disclosure of the risks and comprehensive and accessible communication of the associated information. The final acceptance of the risk may then depend on people's confidence in the risk management procedures that are proposed.

### 3.6. *Monitoring and Surveillance*

The third objective of HIA is the management of the health risks associated with the project under study. This phase starts with the conclusions of the EIS, where the basis of a health risk management is discussed, continues with the permitting procedure following the EIA, but is put into practice when the project is operational. Therefore, it is absolutely essential, during the post project evaluation phase, to find out whether the proposed mitigating measures are either implemented or effective.

An overview of the critical steps in integrating health in EIA is provided in Figure 26. The figure indicates, as described above, that scoping, submission of ToR, the EIS preparation itself, the public participation phases and the post project analysis are, in particular, the main procedural steps in which distinct HIA actions need to be taken.

## 4. Conclusions

Health effects of waste management policies will also remain a main issue of concern throughout the next century. Disposing of all forms of waste, with an ever-increasing variety of products and in ever-increasing amounts, will remain a constant challenge for society. There are in practice, currently, relatively few choices for routes of disposal available: essentially landfill and incineration. Composting, recycling, re-use, and definitely prevention are attractive theoretical and environmentally highly desirable options, but have limited influence on the amounts of waste which are managed today.

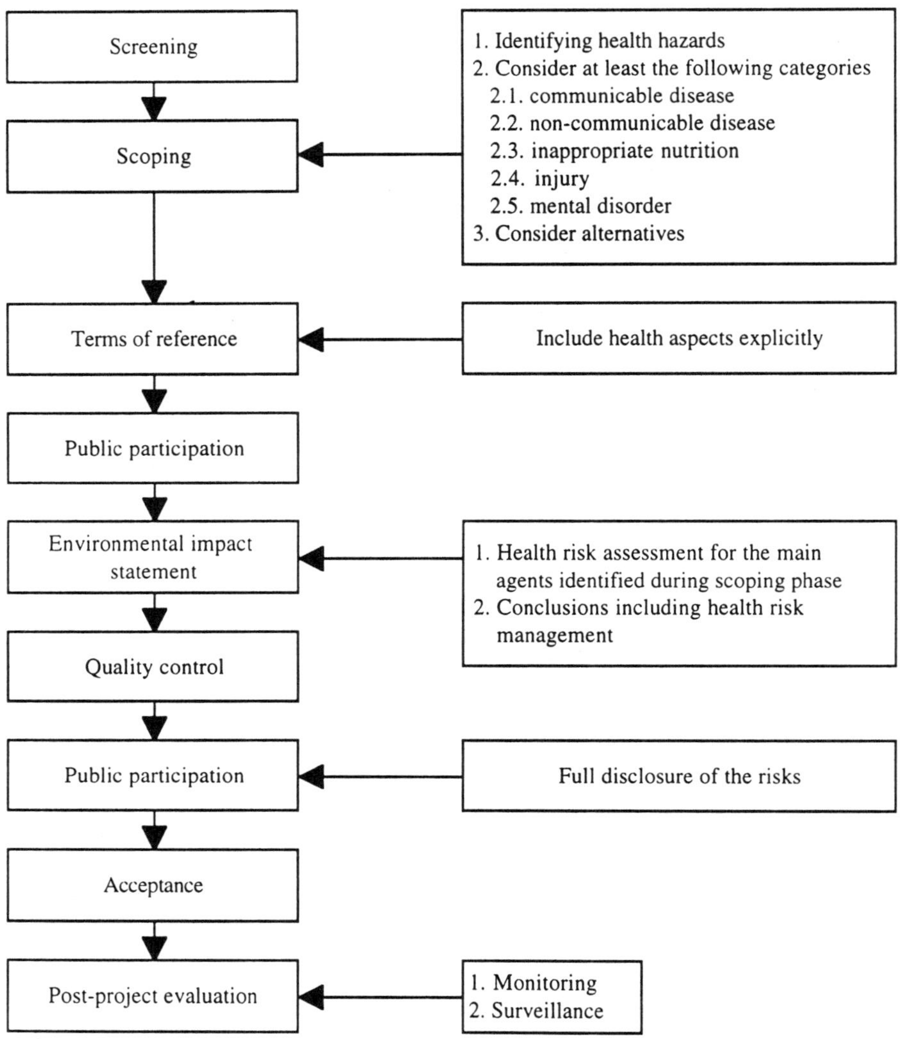


*Figure 26.* A standard EIA procedure. Indicated are the specific health issues to be incorporated into the different procedural steps.

Major concerns over landfill stem from the leachate which contaminates the groundwater, and the landfill sites as such, which show up as black dots on each soil contamination map. Air pollution arising from waste incinerators has become an important issue. Objections to incineration have to do not only with theoretical considerations but also with the impressive record of poorly-equipped and badly-managed installations emitting technically unacceptable and for health, highly undesirable, amounts of pollutants.

This context also allows for the prediction that, in the future, decision-makers and society at large will ask questions not only about the health impacts of the actual plants, but also about the projects which will be realised in the future.

Waste deposit sites, waste incinerators and other industrial facilities for waste management are subject to EIA. HIA is the most appropriate methodology which is available to respond to the questions people have on possible health consequences. HIA is, however, also characterised by important limitations. These are the main ones:

- Hazard identification is, by nature, a **post-factum** activity. One identifies hazards of situations which existed in the past. Therefore, the impact of the results on prospective approaches as EIA will always be limited;

- In both hazard and risk identification, there is a chronic **lack of knowledge**. Even for a debated issue and intensively-studied group of chemicals such as dioxins, we hardly have the instruments today to quantify the carcinogenic effects. On the other, hand there are actually no data available to quantify the immunologic, reproduction or neurotoxicity hazard;

- In most countries, EIA legislation does not require follow-up, **monitoring and surveillance**. Therefore these follow-up activities are simply not done. This puts an important burden on the effectiveness and efficiency of EIA. Moreover, further investments are required, to improve monitoring technology and early warning diagnostics.

It is imperative to erode, and where possible to remove, these obstacles to a high-quality HIA. This is, however, only possible when working on:

- outspoken national policies for environment and health;
- more and well-targeted research;
- improved design and scientifically higher-standard conduct of HIA within EIA;
- evidence-based decision-making;
- improved education and training on these issues.

It should be noted that these coincide with the objectives of ASPIS.

Even when this progress is realised, the overview of the health effects summarised in Tables 39 to 42 of the concluding chapter, show that in many situations health risks cannot be quantified. In these cases HIA does not apply. It is important to recognise implicitly this main limitation of HIA. In such cases the precautionary principle applies.

## References

Adang, D., and De Stordeur, H. (1996) Milieuzorg in Nederlandse en Vlaamse gezondheidszorginstellingen, MSc. Thesis, Human Ecology Department, Vrije Universiteit Brussel, Belgium. (in Dutch)

BMA - British Medical Association (1998) *Health and Environmental Impact Assessment*, Earthscan Publications Ltd., London.

Buekens, A., De Caevel, B., and Neyt, A. (1999) Risk analysis, in B. Nath, L. Hens, P. Compton and D. Devuyst (eds), *Environmental Management in Practice*, Routledge, London and New York, pp. 144-168.

Dolk, H., Vrijheid, M., Armstrong, B., Abramsky, L., Bianchi, F., Garne, E., Nelen, V., Robert, E., Scotte, Y.E.S., Stone, D., and Terconi, R. (1998) Risk of congenital anomalies near hazardous-waste landfill sites in Europe: the Eurohazon study, *The Lancet* **152**, 423-427.

Hens, L. (1993) Environmental pollution and risk assessment, in T. Sugahara, K. Torizuka, S. Kobayashi, and Y. Ishii (eds), *Health Risks: Perspectives and Research*, Proceedings of the Fukui Workshop, Health Research Foundation, Kyoto, Japan, pp. 139-171.

Janssens, P., and Hens, L. (1995) Environmental Health Impact Assessment in Flanders, Belgium, *Environmental Management and Health* **6**, 32-37.

Johnston, P., Stringer, R., Santillo, D., and Howard, C.V. (1999) Hazard, exposure and ecological risk assessment, in B. Nath, L. Hens, P. Compton and D. Devuyst (eds), *Environmental Management in Practice*, Routledge, London and New York, pp. 169-187.

Walker, A. (1991) Waste disposal: a fresh look at a rotting problem, *BMJ* **303**, 1391-1394.

Zaponi, G.A. (1989) Methods for the health component of EIA of industrial development projects, *Proceedings of the 10th International Seminar on EIA and Management*, University of Aberdeen, Scotland, 9-22 July.

# CAN ECOLOGICAL TAXES PLAY A ROLE IN DIMINISHING THE HEALTH IMPACTS OF WASTE MANAGEMENT?

C. STEENWEGEN
*AMINAL*
*Graaf De Ferraris Bldg. 3th floor*
*Emiel Jacqmainlaan 156 bus 8*
*B-1000 Brussels*
*BELGIUM*

## Summary

The best way to diminish the health impacts of waste management is to prevent their generation. Economic instruments and in particular environmental taxes can play an important role in such a preventative policy. They allow the scarcity of environmental resources and the external costs related to the generation and management of waste to reflect on the market price system. Environmental taxes in waste management can also be used to discourage the least desirable disposal practices, to fill the cost gap between recovery and disposal, and to prevent society on the whole from bearing the negative consequences of environmentally unfriendly treatment and disposal practices, which is in contradiction to the 'polluter pays' principle. The use of environmental taxes is reasonably practised in a number of EU member states. Most taxes in waste management are either contributions for a community service (like the collection of municipal waste) or taxes on disposal in order to make separate collection and recycling more attractive.



*P. Nicolopoulou-Stamati et al. (eds.), Health Impacts of Waste Management Policies,* 199–213.

In Belgium a set of ecotaxes on products was introduced to support a policy of waste prevention. These taxes are regulatory taxes, which means that their main purpose is to change the behaviour of producers and consumers. Taxes were introduced on one-way beverage containers, throw-away products, industrial packaging, etc. There was a lot of resistance towards the implementation of these taxes. It illustrates that there is a big difference between supporting environmental taxes in theory and in practice.

## 1. More Prevention Leads to Less Negative Health Impacts

Possible health impacts of waste management occur once there is waste. Waste that has to be recycled or disposed of will, in both cases, have possible negative health effects. The best way to avoid negative health effects is to avoid and to prevent waste. This coincides with the official hierarchy in waste management where prevention is preferred to recycling and recycling before disposal. In reality, however, most policies show the opposite order. Prevention of waste involves a change in behaviour on the part of both producers and consumers that must lead to other products. Environmental taxes can play an important role in developing a product policy that is focused on change in consumer behaviour towards certain products (Jacobs and Steenge, 1990).

Historically, environmental policies started with the regulation of the working conditions within a company. Improvement of these working conditions focused for instance on atmospheric standards. During the '70s and '80s attention was given to the environment outside industrial sites: water and air pollution control led to investments in treatment. But one can very well imagine a plant which is managed well, has very strict internal working standards and controls the wastewater and air pollution streams, but produces products which pose an environmental threat when they are used (consumed) or when they finally become useless and become waste. Therefore, the next step in environmental policy is the development of a product policy. Authorities will encourage or discourage the use of some products, because of their environmental properties. In order to achieve this, other policy instruments than those used up to now will be needed (Steenwegen, 1993a).

In this paper, arguments are provided as to why economic instruments can be helpful in order to develop the policy towards products. They have some advantages over the more traditional policy instruments. One of the economic instruments used is ecological taxation. There are all kinds of ecological taxes. It is important that the purpose of the tax is very well determined so that the tax can be chosen in a way that serves the desired purpose. The paper goes into more detail concerning the system of ecological taxes on products which was introduced in Belgium in 1993.

## 2. From Regulatory to Economic Instruments

The proposal to impose taxes on pollution is not new. It was put forward at the turn of the century by the famous British economist Arthur Cecil Pigou. Reflecting on the famous London fogs, Pigou observed that pollution imposed uncovered costs on third parties which were not included in ordinary market transactions. His proposal was to tax pollution by means of a so-called externality tax in order to internalise the damages caused by pollution in ordinary market transactions. While Pigou was a founder of welfare economics in many ways and thus an important source of inspiration for the subsequent welfare state, the external tax was at this time regarded as a rather academic approach to the control of pollution, and did not serve any practical purpose (Andersen, 1995).

Today, the instruments that environmental policies use are traditionally divided into three groups: regulatory instruments (standards, permits, ...), cultural instruments (awareness-raising, education, ...) and economic instruments (subsidies, taxes, ...). Traditionally, the focus is on regulatory instruments. But their use is insufficient to deal with the rapidly changing knowledge about pollution problems. They are too static. During the last decade, economic instruments have become more prominent. They are supposed to have some advantages over regulatory instruments, and more and more authorities realise that an effective policy needs a mix of instruments, which also includes economic instruments and environmental taxes in particular.

## 3. Advantages of Economic Instruments and Taxes (Andersen, 1995; SERV, 1992; European Commission, 1996; De Savornin Lohman, 1990)

Economic instruments have some advantages as compared to regulatory instruments.

- They do not prescribe specific technologies or solutions, but leave it to the target groups to decide.
  In contrast, permits not only contain emission levels to be reached, but also often stipulate how these permitted levels should be reached (what kind of technology should be used, what kind of treatment should be installed, ...). More and more, the conviction is growing that the target groups themselves often have more knowledge about possible solutions than the authorities. Using taxes allows the target groups to decide upon the technical or managerial options of their preferences.

- They allow for more efficient ways of dealing with non-point sources of pollution which cannot be controlled by permits.
  In the past, environmental policies focused mainly on point sources (factories, electricity plants, incinerators, ...). However, diffuse pollution is as important and much more difficult to control because it is pollution that is most of the time connected to the end-use (the consumption) of products (pesticides, cars, electrical equipment, etc.). To deal with diffuse pollution, instruments are needed which have an impact on the consumption phase of products. Economic instruments are such instruments.

- They ensure that control of pollution takes place where the marginal costs are lowest, thus ensuring substantial cost-savings.
  For some industries it takes a lot more effort and means to reach a particular standard than for others. Using similar permits and standards for all of them, marginal costs will be too high. By using an economic instrument such as an ecological tax, every company can make its own cost-profit analysis and act accordingly.

- Contrary to a fixed license, they provide a constant incentive to reduce emissions, and are as such a more dynamic instrument.

It is commonly found that industries are prepared to reach the emission reduction levels authorities ask for, but if not forced by legislation, they will not perform better. Why should they? It does not provide any advantage. On the contrary, it often means more investments. Economic instruments entail the incentive which stimulates industry to keep on moving.

- Because of these dynamics they cause more innovations and force the development of new and cleaner technologies.
  Industries will not only be stimulated to reduce their emissions further than legally needed, but, because they see economic profit in bringing down emissions as far as possible (with reasonable expenses), they will be stimulated to develop new and cleaner technologies (and to use them).

- They generate revenue, sometimes in substantial amounts, revenue which can be used for environmental or other purposes.
  If authorities think about economic instruments and environmental taxes they think especially about the revenue. Since environmental policies are focused on changes in production and consumption changes that need a lot of means, it is possible to speed up the change by using the collected revenues for the environmental policies one would like to develop.

Examples of economic instruments are tradeable permits, deposit-refund systems, taxes and levies. Environmental taxes can be the key to the integration of environmental considerations into a wide array of policy-areas, and this integration is a key to sustainable development.

Environmental taxes differ:

- Depending on the place within the process:
  * at the 'input' side (a tax on resources),
  * at the 'output' side (a product tax),
  * at the effects level (an emission tax),
  * at the production process itself (a process tax).

To determine the best place to localise a tax, it is important to define the environmental goal and the effects the tax should result in.

- Depending on the main goal of the tax, one aims at defining:
  * a regulatory tax

  The main goal of the tax is to shift the behaviour of target groups. The change in behaviour limits the pollution or even prevents it from occurring. If a regulatory tax is effective, target groups will avoid paying it and so the possible revenues will decrease or even not be generated. But they will not be needed since there will be no need to pay for the means to clean up pollution afterwards.
  * a financing tax

  The main goal of the tax is to generate revenue. The basic idea is that environmental policies will cost money anyway, because of historic pollution, continuing pollution, etc. By taxing the activities that an authority considers to be polluting, the principle 'the polluter pays' is put into practice and revenue is generated that can be used to clean up.

In reality, any tax will be a mixture of both. But it is clear that the logic behind them might be very different. Therefore it is important for authorities to decide what the main goal of the taxes will be.

## 4. Environmental Taxes within the EU

The use of economic instruments and taxes is supported by the European Commission (European Commission, 1994; 1996). The Fifth Action Programme on the Environment of the European Commission promotes the use of economic instruments and taxes in environmental policy. Since economic operators take decisions on the basis of economic considerations, such a policy can have the effect of influencing producers' and consumers' behaviour and directing them towards adopting more environmentally friendly attitudes. Where the price of natural resources is low, more waste is generated; also, where the price of waste disposal is significant, waste generators are likely to avoid these costs by making efforts to reduce the generation of waste. Finally, economic instruments, such as charging products which are neither reusable nor recyclable, are methods which are used in some Member States in order to orient consumers' preference towards other products. The Commission will endeavour to promote the use of economic instruments in the waste sector in accordance with the rules of the internal market.

Economic instruments, particularly environmental taxes, are now part of the policies in many European countries (Norway, Sweden, Denmark, Netherlands, Germany, Belgium, ...). There are taxes on resources (sand, chalk, minerals), packaging and disposable products, oil products (gasoline, mineral oils), other energy carriers (coal, electricity, gas, LPG), fertilisers and pesticides, and emissions of $SO_2$, $NO_x$ (Table 24).

*Table 24.* Selected examples of taxes as they are or were used in European countries (SERV, 1993).

| | |
|---|---|
| Denmark | Sand, chalk and minerals, CFC's, one-way beverage containers, throw-away plates, glasses, forks, knives and spoons, packaging of chemicals, gasoline, heavy fuel, light fuel, electricity, coal |
| Germany | Packaging |
| France | Oils |
| the Netherlands | Mineral oils, LPG, coal, gas, gasoline |
| Norway | Electrical energy, gasoline, heavy fuel, batteries with toxic components, one-way packaging, fertilisers, pesticides, coals |
| Sweden | Motor oils, parafine, gas, kerosene |

## 5. Environmental Taxes and Waste Management

Economic instruments in the waste sector allow the scarcity of environmental resources and the external costs related to the generation and management of waste to be reflected in the market price system (Hoevenagel and Opschoor, 1990).

They may take different forms, such as fiscal measures, financial incentives or deposit-refund schemes, and can play a very considerable role in contributing to the achievement of the different objectives of the waste strategy. They can be used to encourage prevention efforts or to discourage the least desirable disposal practices, to fill the cost gap between recovery and disposal, and to prevent society on the whole from bearing the negative consequences of environmentally unfriendly treatment and disposal practices which is in contradiction to the 'polluter pays principle'.

## 6. Development of Environmental Taxes in Waste Management in Flanders

The region of Flanders, Belgium, provides an example of how waste management policies have developed during the last two decades. In contradiction to the priorities in waste management, as they are internationally accepted, waste management in Flanders, as in many other European countries, was first oriented to the final disposal of the waste and was reoriented afterwards towards recovery and recycling, and finally to prevention. The use of environmental taxes followed this process (Van Humbeeck and Deketelaere, 1994).

### *6.1. 1987: A Tax on Disposal*

In 1987 a tax on the disposal of waste (dumping and incineration) was introduced. Its purpose was to stimulate the municipalities to diminish the ever growing amount of waste that needed to be disposed of. In the beginning the tax rate varied from US$ 0.03 to about US$ 3.00 per ton (for dumping of industrial waste). In the meantime, this system of taxes has changed in many ways. Today, not only is the tax-rate much higher (going up to US$ 20 per ton), but the purpose of the tax has also changed. Purposes today are to stimulate the municipalities:

- to collect the waste separately to make recycling possible;
- to incinerate, instead of dumping;
- to incinerate in an installation with energy recuperation or emissions treatment installation instead of in an installation without one of those.

The tax rates are determined in such a way that the price incentives are clear:

- separate collection is not more expensive than disposal;
- incineration is less expensive than dumping;
- incineration with either emission treatment or energy recuperation is less expensive than without;

- incineration with both purification and energy recuperation is the cheapest.

The result is that there is an important shift towards cleaner disposal and more recovery and recycling. But another result is that the cost of waste management for the municipalities increases dramatically.

### 6.2. *1992: A Tax on Products* (Defeyt *et al.*, 1992)

From 1987 on, the conditions for dumping and incinerating became more severe and the tax rates increased, but this did not change the trend of ever increasing amounts of waste. For the municipalities and the regions it meant that the price for waste management increased dramatically.

In an effort to orient waste policies in Belgium from recycling towards prevention, a law on environmental product taxes was passed by Parliament in 1992. These taxes were in line with three criteria:

1. The main goal of the tax is regulatory and not financial, which explains the high tax rates. These rates are high enough to force producers and consumers to shift towards other products. This means that, even as the taxes are imposed, the market will probably adapt and revenue will be scarce to non-existent.

2. For every product which is subject to an environmental tax, there has to be an environmentally acceptable alternative product for the consumers. If not, producers can just make their products more expensive and consumers have to pay the extra price without their having any possibility of avoiding this. That can be the purpose of an environmental tax in general (for instance in the case of an energy tax) but it is not the intention of this system.

3. Possible and temporary revenues should be used for environmental policies. Although this connection is not necessary, connecting environmental taxes with the development of an environmental policy using the revenues will be more easily accepted by the people.

The most important principles that were included in this ecotax legislation were:

- The tax was an instrument in a policy of prevention. A preventive policy was preferred to the more expensive cleaning-up of the pollution.
- The ecotax was not intended to raise revenue. Instead, the producers of the taxed products were supposed to avoid the tax through a change in behaviour.
- Conditions for exemptions focused on prevention: re-use of packaging, avoidance of throw-away products, decreasing use of pesticides, etc.
- A high tax rate was coupled with conditions for exemption that could be met by companies which had the favoured products already on the market, or which were willing to make an effort to adapt their company's strategy.
- To have a strong incentive for the companies to change behaviour, each company had to meet its specific targets. In this way, it was possible to reward companies which adapted to the new targets and to punish the others which did not wish to match the environmental targets by taxing them.
- To avoid taxes being masked by the market-price, the fact that a product was taxed and the amount of the tax had to be announced on the taxed product in an explicit way. This was a clear signal from the authorities that the use of these labelled products was discouraged. And it prevailed upon the consumers to play their role.
- Every time an ecotax was introduced, the government was supposed to inform the public of the reasons why it chose to discourage the use of a particular product and the recommended alternative.
- An expert commission was installed to follow up on the introduction of these product taxes, which were new among the Belgian policy instruments.

In the meantime, the law changed several times. Today, not much is left of these original principles (Opvolgingscommissie betreffende de milieutaksen, 1994; 1995; 1996):

- No more room for preventive measures. The preference for re-use was abandoned and the focus was moved towards recycling.
- Measures targeted towards individual companies were replaced by collective systems, omitting incentives to invest and adapt. It is useful to point out that this happened under strong pressure from the industrial sectors to whom the tax applied.
- The consumer was also left out. There is no clear sign on the taxed products, and there are no campaigns to inform the people.

A few examples comparing the original set-up with the way the taxes were finally implemented might clarify this shift in principles:

- Beverage containers:
  * originally: exemption for a company if 60-90 per cent reusables on the market;
  * implemented: exemption for the whole sector if 60-90 per cent is collected and recycled;
  * lost: the aim to shift from one-way to reusable. The aim to use the 'first mover' advantage for companies that want to make the shift.
- Batteries:
  * originally: exemption for a company if deposit-refund system, that was able to collect up to 90 per cent of the used batteries, was installed;
  * implemented: a collective collection system paid for by the consumer when buying the battery, independent of whether it is returned or not;
  * lost: the aim to give the consumer the role of collecting the batteries instead of throwing them away.
- Pesticides:
  * originally: about 400 pesticides were taxed depending on their (eco)toxicity. The most toxic ones got a tax so high that they would be priced out of the market. The less toxic ones were taxed so that consumers were stimulated to use less of shift to even less toxic ones.
  * implemented: 3 pesticides were taxed, but exempted if their market-share went down over time. All the others were exempted.
  * lost: the aim of considerably diminishing the use of pesticides overall and more specifically the more (eco)toxic ones.

## 7. Introduction and Implementation of Environmental Taxes: from Theory to Practice (Aelvoet and Steenwegen, 1992; Steenwegen, 1993b)

In Belgium, an interesting experience in introducing environmental taxes has shown some remarkable aspects of this type of introduction, but should be kept in mind by whoever wants to use this instrument:

- Economic instruments enjoy a high degree of support from the public and other target groups like industry sectors, and government bodies as long as they remain theory.

- There is an important difference between supporting the use of economic or more market-oriented instruments in general, and the attitude towards specific environmental taxes.
- When it comes to the choice of environmental taxes, those who will have to bear the costs of the intervention often have strong incentives to lobby against particular measures.
- The potentially taxed group can provide policy-makers with very specific and detailed information to prove that this tax is unjustified and does not serve the environmental goal.
- Since policy-makers often lack information on the way a tax should be designed or its possible impact, they depend to a high degree on the information provided by the target groups.
- Once decision on a tax has been taken in principle, the next step for target groups is to lobby for exemptions.
- The tax rate in itself is a difficult issue and will often become subject to negotiations. There are several methods to determine the rate of ecological taxes:
    * One possibility is to determine the external costs one wants to internalise. This is, however, often difficult. That is probably the reason why those who feel threatened by ecotaxes favour this approach. They hope it will take a long time to figure it all out, and in the meantime, there is no tax.
    * Another possibility is to make sure that the desired change of behaviour takes place. This is of course easier to realise. The elasticity of a product can give an answer to the question on how the consumers will react to a different price for a particular product. If the elasticity is not known, a system of trial and error by which a tax rate is changed can be used.

  In Belgium, the second approach was followed.
- An environmental tax on products is designed by the Ministry of Finance and not by the Ministry of Environment. The Ministry of Finance's first interest is to generate (relatively stable and predictable) revenue.
- Tax ministries prefer administrative simplicity and feasibility. Yet many environmental problems are complex and require a creative tax design.
- It is easier to adapt the existing tax-system than to introduce new taxes. Screening the existing tax-system helps to eliminate existing taxes or tax-exemptions that are contradictory to a better environment.

## 8. **Life Cycle Analysis** (Idenburg and Steenge, 1990; Vollebergh, 1991)

A preventive waste policy which aims at preventing the generation of waste must begin with the product and production process. Waste management concerns have to be fully taken into account from the product's design or conception phase. To be effective, it implies that action is necessary at all stages of a product's life cycle from production, use, collection, re-use, recycling to final disposal. Producers, material suppliers, trade, consumers and public authorities share specific waste management responsibilities. However it is the product manufacturer who has a predominant role. The manufacturer decides on the waste management potential of his product through design, conception, use of specific materials, composition of the product and its marketing. Authorities must decide which products are allowed onto the market and which are not for ecological reasons. How can a government, how can public authorities judge a product? How can they decide which product is environmentally preferable and which one is not? If we want to develop a product policy, we need instruments to do so. Today, an existing instrument is Life Cycle Analysis (LCA). An LCA aims at looking at a product throughout its complete life cycle and assessing the environmental impact in the different stages of this life cycle (the cradle to grave approach). Although these LCAs give very valuable information on the products concerned, they are too static to evaluate the highly dynamic development of products and product groups (insiders thus speak of LCPs (Life Cycle Paralysis) instead of LCAs). It is necessary to keep on thinking of other ways to ecologically evaluate products.

## 9. Conclusions

Economic instruments and environmental taxes are dynamic instruments. There is some practice in several EU-member states, but more practice is needed to avoid the poor use or design of this policy instrument. This will (partly) be a process of trial and error.

Environmental taxes can be used in waste management. They can have different goals, varying from discouraging irresponsible disposal to stimulating waste prevention. The implementation of taxes is always a difficult exercise. Environmental taxes are not exempt from this common rule. The authority that tries to implement these taxes (especially taxes on products) can expect a lot of resistance coming from almost all those involved. The purpose and the possible impacts of a tax are matters of sound thinking.

## References

Aelvoet, M., and Steenwegen, C. (1992) De politieke strijd rond de invoering van de ecotaks. Een getuigenis, in *Political Yearbook of Belgium*, Res Publica, Brussels, pp. 445-457. (in Dutch)

Andersen, M.S. (1995) The use of economic instruments for environmental policy - a half hearted affair, http://www.iisd.ca/linkages/consume/skou.html.

Defeyt, P., Van Hecke, J., Busquin, Ph., Vandenbroucke, F., Poncelet, J.-P., Van Grembergen, P., Aelvoet, M., and Simons, H. (1992) Voorstel van Bijzondere Wet tot wijziging van de Bijzondere Wet van 16 januari 1989 betreffende de financiering van de Gemeenschappen en de Gewesten, Kamer stuk 604/1 – 91/92. (in Dutch)

De Savornin Lohman, A.F. (1990) Haken en ogen aan de ekotaks, in *Ekonomische Statistische Berichten*. (in Dutch)

European Commission - EC (1994) Fifth Action Programme.

European Commission - EC (1996) Community Strategy for Waste Management, communication from the Commission on the review of the strategy, COM(96)399 final.

Hoevenagel, R., and Opschoor, J.B. (1990) *Economische waardering van milieuveranderingen: mogelijkheden en beperkingen.* (in Dutch)

Idenburg, A., and Steenge, A.D. (1990) *Environmental policy in single-product and joint production input-output models.*

Jacobs, M., and Levett, R. (1993) Economic instruments and recovery of resources from waste, ERL report, comments, paper presented at the conference of the National Recycling Forum.

Opvolgingscommissie betreffende de milieutaksen (1994) Jaarverslag, Kanselarij van de Eerste Minister, Brussels. (in Dutch)

Opvolgingscommissie betreffende de milieutaksen (1995) Jaarverslag, Kanselarij van de Eerste Minister, Brussels. (in Dutch)

Opvolgingscommissie betreffende de milieutaksen (1996) Jaarverslag, Kanselarij van de Eerste Minister, Brussels. (in Dutch)

Sociaal Economische Raad voor Vlaanderen - SERV (1992) *Het economisch instrumentarium inzake milieubeleid.* (in Dutch)

Sociaal Economische Raad voor Vlaanderen – SERV (1993) *Sociaal-economische implicaties van de invoering van milieutaksen.* (in Dutch)

Steenwegen, C. (1993a) Het ecotaks-akkoord, een eerste stap in een productbeleid? *Leefmilieu* **16** (**2**), 64-69. (in Dutch)

Steenwegen, C. (1993b) Het rare verhaal van de milieuheffingen en de ecotaksen, in R. Willems (ed.) *Milieujaarboek 1993*, VUB Press, Brussels, pp. 157-176. (in Dutch)

Van Humbeeck, P., and Deketelaere, K. (1994) *Milieufiscaliteit, suggesties voor de ontwikkeling van een algemene beleidsvisie.* (in Dutch)

Vollebergh, H.R.J. (1991) Vervuilen schaadt, betalen baat, in *Economische Statistische Berichten.* (in Dutch)

# CO-ORDINATED REGIONAL ACTION FOR THE REDUCTION OF SOLID WASTE POLLUTION IN THE FRAMEWORK OF THE MEDITERRANEAN ACTION PLAN

G. KAMIZOULIS
*WHO/EURO Project Office*
*Mediterranean Action Plan*
*Vassileos Konstantinou 48*
*11635 Athens*
*GREECE*

## Summary

Urban solid waste can affect the pollution of the sea in a number of ways: through the release of raw waste into the sea, directly or indirectly, especially plastics, and through emissions into the atmosphere of pollutants which may be generated by the combustion of these waste products. For the reduction in pollution reaching the Mediterranean Sea, the riparian states will consider relevant targets and regional activities which include *inter alia* measures related to urban solid wastes. The proposed targets are: (1) by the year 2025 at the latest, to base urban solid waste management on reduction at source, separate collection, recycling, composting and environmentally sound disposal, and (2) by the year 2005 at the latest, to base urban solid waste management on reduction at source, separate collection, recycling, composting and environmentally sound disposal in all cities and urban agglomerations exceeding one hundred thousand inhabitants and areas of concern. The proposed activities at regional level are: (1) by the year 2000 to formulate and adopt guidelines for environmentally suitable and economically feasible systems of



*P. Nicolopoulou-Stamati et al. (eds.), Health Impacts of Waste Management Policies*, 215–222.

collection, including separate collection, and disposal of urban solid waste; and (2) by the year 2005, to develop programmes for the reduction and recycling of urban solid waste.

## 1. Introduction

The riparian States of the Mediterranean Sea, conscious of the economic, social, health and cultural value of the marine environment of the Mediterranean Sea Area, recognising the threat posed by pollution to the marine environment, and mindful of the special hydrographic and ecological characteristics of the Mediterranean Sea Area and its particular vulnerability to pollution, agreed in 1975 to launch an Action Plan for the Protection and Development of the Mediterranean Basin (MAP) and, in 1976, to sign a Convention for the Protection of the Mediterranean Sea against Pollution (Barcelona Convention).

The Contracting Parties to the Barcelona Convention, recognising the danger posed to the marine environment, living resources and human health by pollution from land-based sources and activities, and the serious problems resulting therefrom in many coastal waters and river estuaries of the Mediterranean Sea, primarily due to the release of untreated, insufficiently treated or inadequately disposed of domestic or industrial discharges, and desirous of adapting the Mediterranean Action Plan, Barcelona Convention and their protocols to the development of the environmental international law, to the United Nations Conference on Environment and Development (Rio de Janeiro, 1992), adopted in Barcelona in 1995 phase II of the Action Plan for the protection of the marine environment and sustainable development of the coastal areas of the Mediterranean as well as substantial amendments to the Convention and their Protocols. Furthermore, in Syracuse in 1996 a new revised Protocol for the Protection of the Mediterranean Sea against Pollution from Land-Based Sources and Activities (LBS Protocol) was signed, which takes into account the Global Programme of Action for the protection of the marine environment against pollution from land-based activities, adopted in Washington in 1995.

In accordance with the 1996 LBS Protocol, the Contracting Parties agreed to take all appropriate measures to prevent, abate, combat and eliminate, to the fullest possible extent, pollution of the Mediterranean Sea Area caused by discharges from rivers, coastal establishments or outfalls, or emanating from any other land-based sources and activities within their territories, giving priority to the phasing out of inputs of substances that are toxic, persistent and liable to bio-accumulate. To this end, they agreed to elaborate and implement national and regional action plans and programmes, containing measures and timetables for their implementation.

The Strategic Action Programme (SAP) aims at improving the quality of the marine environment by better shared-management of the land-based pollution. SAP also aims at facilitating the implementation by the Contracting Parties of the LBS Protocol. Therefore, it is designed to assist Parties in taking actions individually or jointly within their respective policies, priorities and resources, which will lead to the prevention, reduction, control and/or elimination of the degradation of the marine environment, as well as to its recovery from the impacts of land-based activities. Achievement of the aims of the SAP will contribute to maintaining and, where appropriate, restoring the productive capacity and biodiversity of the marine environment, ensuring the protection of human health, as well as promoting the conservation and sustainable use of marine living resources. Among the specific objectives of the SAP Programme are: (a) formulation of principles, approaches, measures, timetables and priorities for action, and (b) identification of the elements and preparation of guidelines for the formulation of national action plans for the protection of the marine environment from land-based activities.

An analysis of targets and activities is needed to resolve each pollution priority problem. These targets and activities would be national or regional and would be of a legal, institutional or technical nature. Taking into account the Global Programme of Action (Washington, 1995) and the LBS Protocol, the selected categories of substances cover urban environment and industrial development. Large and even medium-size cities pose similar problems and should be studied in an integrated manner. In most cities, the problems of air pollution, the generation, collection and management of solid waste products, the collection and disposal of domestic wastewater and supplies of drinking water are usually made worse by small and medium-size industries located within the cities and by industrial agglomerations on the outskirts, and can severely affect the environment and human health.

On an international scale, priority has been given to toxic persistent and bio-accumulative pollutants (TPBs) because of their effects on human health, biodiversity and the preservation of ecosystems and long-term and long-distance effects. Less attention is paid to other pollutants, such as toxic and non-persistent or not-bio-accumulative substances, suspended solids, biodegradable organic matter and nutrients, because their effects are much more localised and less persistent. These pollutants are generated primarily in large quantities by industries and their discharge into the environment can cause damage to human health, ecosystems, habitats and biodiversity.

Proposed targets include: over a period of ten years, to reduce by 50 percent discharges, emissions and losses of substances that are toxic, persistent and liable to bio-accumulate from industrial installations.

Persistent organic pollutants (POPs) are a set of organic compounds that: (i) possess toxic characteristics, including effects on the function of the endocrine system; (ii) are persistent; (iii) are liable to bio-accumulate; (iv) are prone to long-range transport and deposition; (v) can result in adverse environmental and human health effects at locations near and far from their source. POPs are typically characterised as having low water solubility and high fat solubility. Most POPs are anthropogenic in origin. Anthropogenic emissions, both point and diffuse, are associated with industrial processes, product use and applications, waste disposal, leaks and spills, and combustion of fuels and waste materials. Once dispersed, clean-up is rarely possible. Because many POPs are relatively volatile, their demobilisation and long-distance redistribution through atmospheric pathways often complicate the identification of specific sources.

POPs have long environmental half-lives. Accordingly, successive releases over time result in the continued accumulation and ubiquitous presence of POPs in the global environment.

The primary transport routes into the marine and coastal environment include atmospheric deposition and surface run-off. Regional and global transport is predominately mediated by atmospheric circulation, but also occurs through sediment transport and oceanic circulation. Movements may also occur through a successive migration of short-range movements resulting from a sequence of volatilisation, deposition and revolatisation processes. Due to these transport patterns and chemical characteristics, there is growing evidence of the systematic migration of these substances to cooler latitudes.

The twelve substances identified by the LBS Protocol are organochlorine compounds and can be divided into three groups:

i) pesticides: DDT; Aldrin, Dieldrin, Endrin; Chlordane; Heptachlor; Mirex; Toxaphene; and Hexachlorobenzene;

ii) industrial chemicals: PCBs (polychlorinated biphenyls);

iii) unwanted contaminants: Hexachlorobenzene; Dioxins and Furans.

*Dioxins and Furans*. The terms *dioxins and furans* are used to describe two groups of environmental pollutants: *polychlorinated dibenzo-p-dioxins (PCDD) and polychlorinated dibenzofurans (PCDF)*. Of these two hundred and ten different substances, the real toxins are the 17 isomers with chlorine substituted in the 2,3,7,8 positions, the most toxic is the *2,3,7,8-tetrachlorodibenzo-p-dioxin (2,3,7,8 TCDD)*, the toxicity of the other sixteen compounds are related with the toxicity of this substance.

*Dioxins and furans* have no use as such, but they can be found as contaminants in some products and can be produced in combustion processes. The sources of *dioxins and furans* can be natural or human. Natural sources include forest fires, volcanic eruptions or enzymatic and photolytic reactions. There is no doubt today that the presence of compounds of *dioxins and furans* in the environment occurs primarily as a result of anthropogenic practices.

The most important anthropogenic sources of dioxins and furans are:

i) combustion installations: incineration of urban, industrial and hospital waste, combustion of residual sludges, fossil power plants;

ii) small combustion sources: car engines, domestic heating;

iii) the manufacture and use of certain pesticides, especially *chlorophenoxyacids (2.4-D and 2.4.5-T), chlorinated phenols and PCBs*, in which dioxins and furans are found as impurities;

iv) other processes, such as paper pulp bleaching, the metallurgy of metals, the recovery of metals (mainly copper wire and electric motors and copper and aluminium turnings);

v) accidents: fires involving chlorinated materials, mainly chlorophenols and PCBs.

Proposed targets are: (1) *by the year 2010, to phase out inputs of the nine pesticides and PCBs and reduce to the fullest possible extent inputs of unwanted contaminants: hexachlorobenzene, dioxins and furans;* (2) *by the year 2005, to reduce 50 percent inputs of the priority 12 POPs*, and (3) *by the year 2005, to collect and dispose of all PCB waste in a safe and environmentally sound manner.*

Proposed activities at the Regional level are: (1) to provide Contracting Parties with technical information and advice on the nine pesticides and PCB substitutes and make appropriate recommendations; (2) to develop programmes for sharing and exchanging technical information and advice regarding the environmentally sound disposal of the existing quantities of the nine pesticides and PCBs. These programmes should consider progressive elimination, including the decontamination of equipment and containers; and (3) to prepare guidelines for the application of BEP and if possible BAT at the point sources of dioxins and furans mentioned on the preceding page.

Proposed activities at the National level are: (1) to make, over a period of two years, an inventory of quantities and uses of the nine pesticides and PCBs, as well as of the industries which manufacture or condition them; (2) by the year 2000, to phase out the use of the nine pesticides, except those uses which involve the safeguarding of human life when the latter is in danger or when a risk/benefit analysis is very conclusive, according to WHO recommendations; (3) by the year 2000, to prohibit the manufacture, trade and new use of PCBs and, by the year 2010, to ban all existing uses of PCBs; (4) to prepare pilot programmes aimed at the safe disposal of the PCBs; these programmes should consider progressive elimination, including the decontamination of equipment and containers; (5) by the year 2000, to organise the collection and environmentally sound disposal of the existing quantities of the nine pesticides; and (6) to reduce the emission of *HCB, dioxins and furans* as much as possible and, in order to do so, to promote the implementation of environmental audits and apply BEP and if possible BAT to the processes which generate these compounds, such as waste-incineration or recovery of metals, mainly copper wire and electric motors.

## 2. Conclusions

### *2.1. Proposed Targets*

- By the year 2025 at the latest, to base urban solid waste management on reduction at source, separate collection, recycling, composting and environmentally sound disposal.

- By the year 2005 at the latest, to base urban solid waste management on reduction at source, separate collection, recycling, composting and environmentally sound disposal in all cities and urban agglomerations exceeding one hundred thousand inhabitants and areas of concern.

### *2.2. Proposed Activities at Regional Level*

- By the year 2000, to formulate and adopt guidelines for environmentally suitable and economically feasible systems of collection, including separate collection, and disposal of urban solid waste.

- By the year 2005, to develop programmes for the reduction and recycling of urban solid waste.

### *2.3. Proposed Activities at National Level*

- By the year 2000, to develop national plans and programmes for the reduction at source and environmentally sound management of urban solid waste.

- By the year 2005, to establish environmentally suitable and economically feasible systems of collection and disposal of urban solid waste in cities and urban agglomerations of more than one hundred thousand inhabitants.

- To promote the reduction and recycling of urban solid waste.

## References

UNEP (1992) Mediterranean Action Plan and Convention for the Protection of the Mediterranean Sea against Pollution and its related protocols.

UNEP (1995) Global Programme of Action for the Protection of the Marine Environment against Pollution from Land-Based Activities.

UNEP (1997) Mediterranean Action Plan and Convention for the Protection of the Marine Environment and the Coastal Region of the Mediterranean and its Protocols, informal document (revised).

UNEP (1997) Report of the Tenth Ordinary Meeting of the Contracting Parties to the Convention for the Protection of the Mediterranean Sea against Pollution and its protocols.

# CASE STUDIES

# A LOCAL INCREASED INCIDENCE OF OROFACIAL CLEFTS IN AMSTERDAM: THE RESULT OF OPEN COMBUSTION OF CHEMICALS?

G.W. TEN TUSSCHER
G.A. STAM
J.G. KOPPE
*Neonatology Department*
*Emma Children's Hospital/Academic Medical Centre*
*University of Amsterdam*
*PO Box 22660*
*1100 DD Amsterdam*
*THE NETHERLANDS*

## Summary

*Hypothesis:* The open chemical combustions in Zeeburg, Amsterdam, the Netherlands, from the year 1961 up to and including 1969 resulted in a local increased incidence of orofacial clefts during this period.

*Study:* A retrospective observational epidemiological study was performed, comparing the trend of the incidence of non-syndromal orofacial clefts during the sixties for the Zeeburg maternity clinic with that of the Wilhelmina Gasthuis. Both clinics were situated in Amsterdam, but varying in distance and direction from the incineration works. Thereafter, the addresses of the mothers giving birth to infants with orofacial clefts were plotted on a map of Amsterdam.



*P. Nicolopoulou-Stamati et al. (eds.), Health Impacts of Waste Management Policies,* 225–238.

*Results:* Of the eight thousand, eight hundred and three children born in the Zeeburg clinic during this period, twenty-one had a non-syndromal orofacial cleft, producing an average incidence of 2.4 per 1000 births. For the years 1963 through 1965 the incidence rose dramatically to peak at 7.1 per 1000, before plateauing at an average incidence of 1.68 per 1000 births, still 155 per cent higher than in the Wilhelmina clinic (average incidence of 0.66 per 1000 during the years 1966 through 1969). During the ten-year period the Wilhelmina clinic exhibited no such rise. The incidence of non-syndromal orofacial clefts at the Wilhelmina clinic at no time exceeded 2.3 per 1000 births during the ten-year period. The addresses of the mothers of the infants with orofacial clefts in Zeeburg were grouped primarily to the north-west (and a smaller group to the west) of the incineration works.

*Conclusion:* A relation between the open incineration of the chemicals and a local increased incidence of orofacial clefts seems very likely.

## 1. Introduction

While researching an article on epilepsy and congenital defects in 1973, Koppe and her colleagues serendipitously discovered what seemed to be a surprisingly high incidence of orofacial clefts during the 1960's in the Zeeburg area of Amsterdam, the Netherlands. This high incidence was not comparable to the incidence at a maternity clinic (the Wilhelmina Gasthuis) elsewhere in the same city (Koppe, 1973). Much later it was discovered that chemicals had been incinerated in the open air in the vicinity of the Zeeburg maternity clinic, at the Diemerzeedijk, during the 1960's. A coincidence?

From literature sources and our ongoing studies on the possible effects of dioxin exposure on the growth and development of children, we have become aware of the (possible) teratogenic and/or carcinogenic effects of these environmental pollutants. We therefore hypothesised that the local increased incidence of orofacial clefts was a direct result of the open incineration of the chemicals at the Diemerzeedijk incinerator.

### *The Diemerzeedijk Waste Site*

The company responsible for the incineration, which took place from 1961 to 1973, was allocated the 'Diemerzeedijk' terrain in 1961. Commissioning commenced shortly thereafter. It was soon apparent that a tremendous demand existed for such an incinerator, and major multinational companies, many of whom were later to deny the fact, exploited the opportunity in order to dispose of chemical wastes. The incineration must have proved lucrative, for the quantities of incinerated chemicals increased phenomenally. The incineration company promptly began importing waste chemicals for combustion from all over Europe, from countries such as Germany and Czechoslovakia, and even from as far afield as Finland. Scant registration of the quantities incinerated was kept (Table 25). (However, these figures have been shown to be up to seventy percent understated)!

*Table 25.* The quantities of chemicals incinerated at the Diemerzeedijk incinerator, 1960-1973. The quantities up to 1968 have been shown to be up to 70 per cent understated (see text) (DOW GRM, 1987).

| Year | Quantities of incinerated chemicals | Remarks |
|---|---|---|
| 1960 | nil | |
| 1961 | unknown | Terrain allocated to the incineration company |
| 1962 | unknown | |
| 1963 | unknown | |
| 1964 | unknown | Complaints of extreme smells and air pollution |
| 1965 | 4 235 tons | |
| 1966 | 8 574 tons | |
| 1967 | 9 061 tons | Incineration only permitted during south westerly winds |
| 1968 | 11 789 tons | |
| 1969 | unknown | |
| 1970 | 2 500 tons | Under management of the City of Amsterdam |
| 1971 | 2 500 tons | Under management of the City of Amsterdam |
| 1972 | 2 500 tons | Under management of the City of Amsterdam |
| 1973 | Cessation | Cessation of incineration activities |

While the rapidly increasing activities were probably favourable to the exploiters, this was not so for many residents of the surrounding urban areas. Innumerable complaints regarding the extreme smells and air pollution were made. Whilst the incinerations (one to three thousand tons per time) took place merely once every one to three months, it was noted that on the days that they took place, sedimentation powders fell over the surrounding areas. This was more than likely also a consequence of the manner of incineration: the 100-litre drums of chemicals were lined up, in lines of at times more than a hundred metres long, tens of metres wide and eight to ten barrels high. A number of the drums were then pierced, allowing the contents to flow out and this was then ignited. According to the official report of the City of Amsterdam (DOW GRM, 1987) this was quite an impressive scene to witness, with drums flying high into the sky as the chemicals and drums exploded! The thick, pitch-black smoke columns, more than 100 metres high, were visible from tens of kilometres away. The fire department was notified before the chemicals were ignited.

The incineration company was found to be in violation of environmental legislation during the years of operation. This eventually led to the City of Amsterdam taking over the responsibility and drastically reducing the number of incinerations, and finally decommissioning the waste site in 1973.

Since then, the site has been found to contain numerous toxic chemicals and in toxic concentrations. In 1998, a quarter of a century after its closure, the Diemerzeedijk complex remains a prohibited area - this as a result of the toxicity. Anglers are prohibited from fishing in the vicinity of the Diemerzeedijk, for fear of their possible ingestion of the contaminated aquatic biota.

## 2. Method

Analysing possible environmental influences on the health and well-being of individuals has, in the past, proven a difficult challenge. With the advent of modern technological advances, many occupational health hazards have been plotted. For the 'uncontained, unisolated' environment this has been more problematic, and animal studies, while indicative, are not perfect, because of well documented interspecies variations (Bracken, 1997). It was therefore decided to test the clinical observation by way of a retrospective observational epidemiological study. The trend of the incidence of orofacial clefts at the

Zeeburg maternity clinic for the period from 1960 up to and including 1969 was compared with the quantities of combusted chemicals during this same period. Thereafter the trends of the incidence of orofacial clefts were compared at two maternity clinics in Amsterdam, the Netherlands, over the ten-year period from 1960 up to and including 1969. Finally the addresses of the mothers who gave birth to children with orofacial clefts were plotted on a map of Amsterdam

All the pregnancies at a maternity clinic in Zeeburg, Amsterdam, the Netherlands, situated near the waste incinerator mentioned above were reviewed from the medical log books. Each pregnancy was sufficiently documented. The number of orofacial clefts was noted. In order to exclude syndromal clefts, other abnormalities were also noted, as were specifics such as gender. These data were then related to the total number of births, live and still-born.

The same procedure was performed for another maternity clinic, Wilhelmina Gasthuis, also situated in Amsterdam, the Netherlands, yet in the west of the city, about 12 km away from the waste incinerator (the wind in the Netherlands is mostly from the south-west).

It is important to note that births in the Zeeburg clinic were on social indications only; for example, for mothers who had no appropriate room at home for the delivery. Any pathologic pregnancies were sent to the Wilhelmina clinic, where specialised centres for mother and child were available. The Wilhelmina clinic births were thus both on social and on pathological indication.

## 3. Results

From a total of eight thousand, eight hundred and three births in Zeeburg, in the period from 1 January 1960 up to and including 31 December 1969, twenty-two babies had a non-syndromal orofacial cleft (Table 26). Thus an average incidence of 2.5 per 1000 births. In 1963, nine hundred and seventy-three infants were born in Zeeburg, of which five had an orofacial cleft, producing an incidence of 5.1 per 1000 births. In Zeeburg in 1964, nine hundred and ninety infants were born, of which no less than seven had an orofacial cleft - an incidence of 7.1 per 1000 births. In the years 1963 and 1964, three and two respectively of the cases of orofacial clefts were of cleft palatum molle (soft palate). The incidence of orofacial clefts for the years 1963 and 1964 were statistically significantly higher for the Zeeburg clinic than for the Wilhelmina clinic.

*Table 26.* The incidence of orofacial clefts at the Zeeburg maternity clinic for the years 1960 up to and including 1969.

| Year | Total no. of births | no. of CLP | no. of CPS | no. of Syndromal cleft | Total no. of clefts | Remarks |
|---|---|---|---|---|---|---|
| 1960 | 894 | 1 | - | | 1 | Sister also had an orofacial cleft |
| 1961 | 996 | 1 | - | - | 1 | Sister also had an orofacial cleft |
| 1962 | 1119 | 1 | - | - | 1 | |
| 1963 | 973 | 2 | 3 | - | 5 | |
| 1964 | 990 | 5 | 2 | - | 7 | |
| 1965 | 860 | 2 | - | - | 2 | |
| 1966 | 758 | 1 | - | - | 1 | |
| 1967 | 929 | - | 1 | 2 | 3 | |
| 1968 | 711 | 1 | 1 | - | 2 | |
| 1969 | 573 | - | 1 | - | 1 | |
| Total | 8803 | 14 | 8 | 2 | 24 | |

CLP = cleft lip with or without cleft palate, CPS = cleft palatum molle (soft palate).

In the maternity clinic Wilhelmina Gasthuis a total of twenty-one thousand and seventy-eight infants were born from 1 January 1960 up to and including 31 December 1969, including twenty-five with a non-syndromal orofacial cleft (Table 27). Therefore the average incidence of orofacial clefts over the ten year period was 1.2 per 1000 births. In 1963 the incidence was 1.0, with two of two thousand one hundred babies born with a non-syndromal orofacial cleft. In 1964, two thousand and eighty-seven infants were born, of which five had an orofacial cleft, producing an incidence of 2.3. At no time during the ten years from 1960 up to and including 1969 did the incidence of infants born with an orofacial cleft rise beyond 3.0 per 1000 births (Figure 27).

*Table 27.* The incidence of orofacial clefts at the Wilhelmina Gasthuis maternity clinic for the years 1960 up to and including 1969.

| Year | Total no. of births | no. of CLP | no. of CPS | no. of Syndromal cleft | Total no. of clefts | Remarks |
|---|---|---|---|---|---|---|
| 1960 | 2364 | 3 | - | 1 | 4 | |
| 1961 | 2353 | 4 | - | 3 | 7 | 1 CLP is sibling of an epilepsy patient |
| 1962 | 2381 | 3 | 1 | - | 4 | |
| 1963 | 2100 | 2 | - | 1 | 3 | |
| 1964 | 2187 | 4 | 1 | - | 5 | |
| 1965 | 2129 | 2 | - | - | 2 | |
| 1966 | 2095 | - | 1 | 1 | 2 | |
| 1967 | 1947 | - | 1 | 1 | 2 | |
| 1968 | 1804 | 2 | - | - | 2 | |
| 1969 | 1718 | 1 | - | 3 | 4 | |
| Total | 21078 | 21 | 4 | 10 | 35 | |

CLP = cleft lip with or without cleft palate, CPS = cleft palatum molle (soft palate).

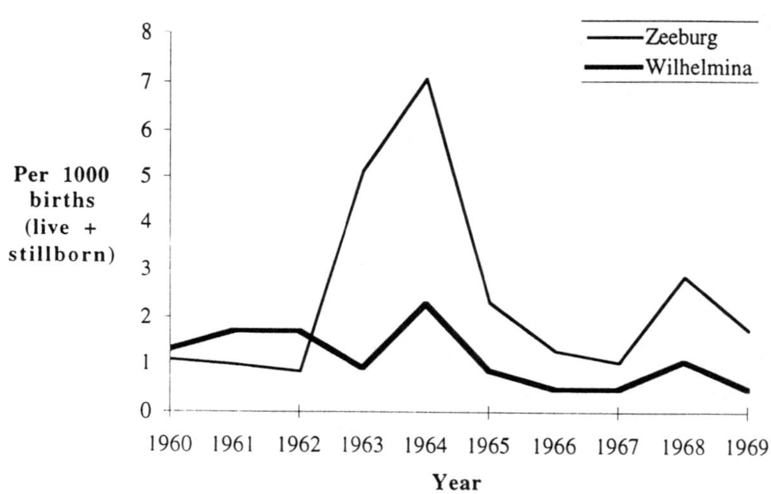


*Figure 27.* The trend of the incidence of orofacial clefts for the Zeeburg and Wilhelmina clinics, for the years 1960 up to and including 1969.

All the addresses of the mothers who gave birth to children with an orofacial cleft were uncovered, with the exception of one of the Zeeburg population and ten of the Wilhelmina population. When the addresses of the children born with an orofacial cleft in the Zeeburg clinic were plotted, there was a remarkable dispersion. No less than fourteen of the twenty-four children were born to mothers living to the north-west of the Diemerzeedijk. There was also a smaller grouping to the west of the incinerator. When the addresses of the children born with an orofacial cleft in the Wilhelmina clinic were plotted, they were far more spread out across the city of Amsterdam, as would be expected.

## 4. Discussion

### *4.1. Comparison*

As Figure 27 graphically illustrates, the incidence of orofacial clefts in the Zeeburg maternity clinic showed a relatively large surge in 1963-64. The atypical trend of incidence over the ten year period, with the peak in 1963-64, was clearly not indicative of the incidence elsewhere in the same city. This can also be seen in Figure 27. The Wilhelmina Gasthuis trend displays an incidence of between 1 and 3 cases per 1000 births. This is in agreement with the average Dutch and Belgian incidence of 1.47 per 1000 births (including both syndromal and non-syndromal clefts) (Derijcke *et al.*, 1996). Furthermore, it is remarkable that the incidence in Zeeburg dropped dramatically during 1965, plateauing at a level 155 per cent higher than the Wilhelmina clinic.

The Zeeburg maternity population was a group selected on optimality regarding favourable, healthy pregnancies, with little chance of pathology. This is in contrast to the Wilhelmina clinic, where the population group was selected on possible or probable pathology. It is therefore to be expected, contrary to what was found, that there would then be a higher incidence of orofacial clefts in the Wilhelmina clinic than in the Zeeburg clinic. This can be seen in the fact that the average incidence of orofacial clefts in the Wilhelmina clinic (1.66 per 1000 births) is higher than the 1.47 per 1000 births reported for the Netherlands (Derijcke *et al.*, 1996).

### *4.2. Airborne pollution*

Research has pointed out that the incineration processes at the Diemerzeedijk incinerator produced large amounts of sedimentation powders, many of which were carried by the wind. Many of the chemicals combusted by the company are known to produce dioxin and dioxin-like sedimentation powders, easily carried by the wind. Eye-witness reports have verified that powdery sedimentations were indeed often seen in the vicinity of the Diemerzeedijk works during incineration (DOW GRM, 1987).

Table 25 shows the registered incinerated chemical quantities from the waste incinerator for the same time period, 1960-73. Incineration activities were only permitted when the wind was blowing from the south-west (DOW GRM, 1987), the reasoning being that any residue would be blown over the IJssel Lake, as opposed to over the urban areas to the south and west of the terrain.

The collected eels and rabbits from the vicinity of the combustion terrain were shown to have toxic concentrations of dioxins in their bodies (DOW GRM, 1987). Additionally, the Dutch Ministry of Water Affairs, in a separate report, concluded that there was an increase in the concentration of PCBs in the neighbouring IJssel Lake (DOW GRM, 1987), and this while bearing in mind that PCBs, due to their hydrophobic nature, are poorly transported by water. Was this increase a result of airborne PCB pollution or due to leakage?

The wind in the Netherlands is normally from the south-west, but often comes from the south-east and east. Assuming that the company only combusted the chemicals while a south-westerly wind was blowing residues and sedimentation powders would then be blown east and north-east, over a lake, the IJssel Lake. What if the wind changed direction during the day, or if the company, in violation of the stipulations, decided to combust while the wind was blowing from the south-east or east? The same residue would then be blown north-west and west over urban areas of Amsterdam. It is then very interesting to find the atypical groupings of orofacial clefts to the north-west and to the west of the Diemerzeedijk incineration complex.

In his overview of the possible health effects of landfill gases, Watson (1998) quoted the British ENTEC report of landfill gases. ENTEC stated that *'in many respects the composition of these community air samples appear similar to the air samples collected from positions immediately above the landfill surface'*. Watson concludes, *'whilst it is not possible to pinpoint the exact mechanism, chemical or combination of chemicals by which the community around a landfill site could be affected there is enough evidence to justify concern'* (Watson, 1998).

It is thus no far-fetched hypothesis to say that a considerable part of north-west Amsterdam was probably polluted by very potent chemicals, and that the residents of Zeeburg were thereby more than likely exposed to toxic concentrations of dioxins. Dioxins are able to pass the placental barrier (Buser, 1985; Hutzinger *et al.*, 1985).

### *4.3. Aetiology*

Orofacial clefts have a multifactorial aetiology. While there has long been evidence of a genetic influence, environmental influences also play a role (Lie *et al.*, 1994). Recently it was postulated that a trend indicated an increased risk of oral clefts with increased overall exposure to glycol ethers, a common industrial and household chemical (Cordier *et al.*, 1997). Additionally, it has been demonstrated that a small yet statistically significant risk of orofacial clefts (especially cleft palates) exists for the offspring of mothers who smoke during the first trimester of their gestation period (Wyszynski *et al.*, 1997; Källén, 1997). The risk increases with increasing exposure, up to 10-fold, when in combination with the gene variant transforming growth factor alpha allele (Shaw *et al.*, 1996). While cigarettes contain many (potentially) toxic substances, it is interesting to note that they also contain N-nitroso compounds and polycyclic aromatic hydrocarbons (for e.g. benzo(a)pyrene). It has been noted that placental oxidation activities, such as the induction of cytochrome P-450 for polycyclic aromatic hydrocarbons, were reduced in malformed infants compared with normal controls, of mothers who smoked during pregnancy (Shaw *et al.*, 1996).

### *4.4. Confounders*

While it is no longer possible to reliably control for further confounders, it is arguable that this is not needed. While smoking in the 1960's was not widespread amongst women in the Netherlands, the Zeeburg clinic population would certainly not have had a greater number of smoking mothers than the Wilhelmina clinic.

This reasoning can also be applied to possible genetic confounders. Neither population was an enclave, and therefore the gene-pools would not have been restricted. While the genetic backgrounds (especially for TGFa) would not be expected to be different for the two populations, any known genetic risk factors would have been indications for delivery in the Wilhelmina clinic.

The socio-economic status of the two populations was similar. Both populations were generally from lower socio-economic groups. This also formed the basis for their social indications for giving birth in a clinic, and not at home - there was no suitable room at home for this purpose.

Furthermore, the use of anti-epileptic drugs could be offered as a possible confounder. A pregnant woman with epilepsy was a pathological condition. Such women would have given birth at the Wilhelmina clinic, and once again, certainly not the Zeeburg clinic. This was also a major reason why Koppe, *et al.*, selected the Zeeburg population as a control group, and the Wilhelmina population as the exposed group in their study on epilepsy and congenital abnormalities (Koppe *et al.*, 1973).

Finally, we must consider vitamin deficiencies. There was a shortage of food in the Amsterdam region, during and after World War II. With respect to calories this was rapidly corrected after the war, but the shortage of folic acid might have lasted longer. Yet, a vitamin deficiency would have meant that the peri-war high incidence of anencephaly would have remained high. To the contrary, the incidence dropped dramatically before and during the sixties, and the socio-economic circumstances improved greatly (Romijn *et al.*, 1983; Romijn *et al.*, 1982). Thus, vitamin deficiencies could not reasonably be offered as an explanation for the extraordinary results.

### *4.5. TCDD effects on palatal formation*

The normal human palate is a result of the fusion of the primary and secondary palatal primordia. This process begins in the fifth embryological week and is completed by the end of the twelfth week, with its most critical period being between the sixth and ninth weeks. Failure to fuse results in an orofacial cleft (Moore and Persaud, 1993). Orofacial cleft anomalies are relatively common with an incidence of 1-2 per 1000 births, with a higher prevalence amongst males than females (Derijcke *et al.*, 1996).

Animal studies with mice elicited cleft palate and hydronephrosis in embryos exposed to TCDD (a dioxin). It was postulated that exposure to a teratogenic dose of TCDD led to disturbed proliferation and differentiation of palatal cells. TCDD is known to bind with the Ah receptor (AhR) and thereby alter transcription of specific genes. AhR is found in palatal epithelial and mesenchymal cells, and has its highest expression in epithelium thereof. Furthermore, AhR mRNA and protein were found to be downregulated in mice palates exposed to TCDD (Abbott, 1995). These studies add credence to the proposed relationship between the open chemical incineration at the Diemerzeedijk incineration complex and the alarming increase in the incidence of orofacial clefts in Zeeburg during the 1960's.

## 5. Conclusions

Let us now summarise what we have found and some of the findings found in a literature search:

1. There were numerous complaints of sedimentation powders as a result of the incineration works.
2. Many of the chemicals combusted are known to produce dioxin- and dioxin-like sedimentation powders when combusted.
3. There was increased PCB concentration found in the IJssel Lake, and eels and rabbits collected from the vicinity of the Diemerzeedijk incineration complex have toxic concentrations of dioxins in their bodies.
4. Dioxins readily pass the placental barrier, collecting in adipose tissues. 2,3,7,8-Tetrachlorodibenzo-p-dioxin, or TCDD, a dioxin, is known to produce hydronephrosis and orofacial clefts in mice. TCDD is known to bind to the aryl hydrocarbon receptor, a receptor seen in high concentrations in epithelial tissues (which also make up the human palate and lip).

5. Chemical agents can cause orofacial clefts; for example, a higher incidence of orofacial clefts was found amongst smoking mothers, mothers exposed to glycol ethers, and the offspring of veterans of the Vietnam war (American and Vietnamese) exposed to the dioxin-based defoliant, Agent Orange.
6. The Zeeburg population was a population selected on optimality regarding health and pregnancy, yet demonstrated an atypical trend and incidence of orofacial clefts for the years from 1960 up to and including 1969.
7. Vitamin deficiencies, smoking mothers, genetic enclaves and anti-epileptica could not reasonably be offered as confounders or an explanation for the abnormal trend and distribution of the orofacial clefts.

In conclusion, while it is probably impossible to prove beyond doubt a cause-effect relationship, the results strongly indicate an association between the open incineration of chemicals, and the increased incidence of orofacial clefts in Zeeburg, Amsterdam, the Netherlands, for the years from 1960 up to and including 1969.

## References


Abbott, B.D. (1995) Review of the interaction between TCDD and glucocorticoids in embryonic palate, *Toxicology* **105**, 365-373.

Bracken, M.B. (1997) Musings on the edge of epidemiology, *Epidemiology* **8** (**4**), 337-339.

Buser, H.R. (1985) Formation, occurrence and analysis of polychlorinated dibenzofurans, dioxins and related compounds, *Environ. Health Perspect.* **60**, 259-267.

Cordier, S., Bergeret, A., Goujard, J., Ha, M.C., Aymé, S., Bianchi, F., Calzolari, E., de Walle, H.E.K., Knill-Jones, R., Candela, S., Dale, I., Dananché, B., de Vigan, C., Fevotte, J., Kile, G., and Mandereau, L. for the Occupational Exposure and Congenital Malformations Working Group (1997) Congenital malformations and maternal occupational exposure to glycol ethers, *Epidemiology* **8** (**4**), 355-363.

Derijcke, A., Eerens, A., and Carels, C. (1996) The incidence of oral clefts: a review, *Br. J. Oral . Maxillofac. Surg.* **34** (**6**), 488-494.

DOW GRM (1987) *Nader Onderzoek Brandplaats Diemerzeedijk*, Opdracht 3930 GRM 33, Amsterdam, Dienst Openbare Werken Bureau Grondmechanica. (in Dutch)

Hutzinger, O., Choudhry, G.G., Chittim, B.G., and Johnston, L.E. (1985) Formation of polychlorinated dibenzofurans and dioxins during combustion, electrical equipment fires and PCB incineration, *Environ. Health Perspect.* **60**, 3-9.

Källén, K. (1997) Maternal smoking and orofacial clefts. *Cleft Palate Craniofac. J.* **34** (**1**), 11-16.

Koppe, J.G., Bosman, W., Oppers, V.M., Spaans, F., and Kloosterman, G.J. (1973) Epilepsie en aangeboren afwijkingen, *Ned. Tijdschr. Geneeskd.* **117** (**6**), 220-224. (in Dutch)

Lie, R.T., Wilcox, A.J., and Skjœrven, R. (1994) A population-based study of the risk of recurrence of birth defects, *N. Engl. J. Med.* **331** (**1**), 1-4.

Moore, K.L., and Persaud, T.V.N. (1993) *The Developing Human*, WB Saunders Company, Philadelphia, London, Toronto, Montreal, Sydney and Tokyo.

Romijn, J.A., Smit, D.E., and Treffers, P.E. (1982) Anencefalie in Nederland in de periode 1950-1980, regionaal en in de tijd, *Ned. Tijdschr. Geneeskd.* **126** (**48**), 2185-2188. (in Dutch)

Romijn, J.A., and Treffers, P.E. (1983) Anencephaly in the Netherlands: a remarkable decline, *The Lancet* **I** (**8314-5**), 64-65.

Shaw, G.M., Wasserman, C.R., Lammer, E.J., O'Malley, C.D., Murray, J.C., Basart, A.M., and Tolarova, M.M. (1996) Orofacial clefts, parental cigarette smoking, and transforming growth factor alpha gene variants, *Am. J. Hum. Genet.* **58** (**3**), 551-561.

Watson, A. (1998) *Possible Health Effects of Landfill Gases*, Presented at the ASPIS Seminar on Health Impacts of Waste Management Policies, Kos, Greece, 12-14 November.

Wyszynski, D.F., Duffy, D.L., and Beaty, T.H. (1997) Maternal cigarette smoking and oral clefts: a meta analysis, *Cleft Palate Craniofac. J.* **34** (**3**), 206-210.

# HEALTH EFFECTS OF A HOUSEHOLD WASTE INCINERATOR NEAR WILRIJK, BELGIUM

N. VAN LAREBEKE
*Department of Radiotherapy, Nuclear Medicine and Experimental Cancerology*
*University of Gent*
*De Pintelaan 185*
*B-9000 Gent*
*BELGIUM*

## Summary

In Wilrijk, Flanders, a cluster of congenital anomalies was discovered amongst inhabitants of the Neerland neighbourhood, situated between the municipal waste incinerator IHK at Edegem (at a distance of about 800 metres) and ISVAG at Wilrijk (at a distance of about 1200 metres). This paper is an overview of the results of health impact studies on these inhabitants during the period 1997-1998. Chromosomal aberrations in peripheral lymphocytes were studied in twenty-four children from Neerland, as compared to twenty children from another neighbourhood in the Antwerp region. No difference was found. Negative confounding might have resulted from the fact that the twenty-four children in the Neerland neighbourhood had six smoking parents, whereas the twenty children in the control group had seventeen smoking parents. The study did not allow for a slight increase in chromosome aberrations. Another study found no difference between the whole of Flanders and the Neerland neighbourhood as to perinatal death. There was, however, a statistically non-significant difference in the incidence of congenital malformations, with an odds ratio of 1.26 (0.80-1.99), confined to children born from



*P. Nicolopoulou-Stamati et al. (eds.), Health Impacts of Waste Management Policies,* 239–250.

parents who had not resided for a long time in Neerland. There was also a statistically significant increase in the number of multiple pregnancies, with an odds ratio of 2.60 (2.08-3.31). Compared to other neighbourhoods in Wilrijk and to Flanders in general, occurrence of failure at school was not increased in Neerland, and there were significantly less children from the Neerland neighbourhood in special education classes. In the third class of maternal school, but not in the first year of maternal school nor in the third year of primary school, allergies and repeated episodes of the common cold were significantly more frequent in children from Neerland than in children from nearby Hemiksem.

It is concluded that although in this population, there is no definitive evidence for the impact of the incinerator emissions on human health, the data are sufficiently indicative to advocate:

- detailed studies on individual exposure and presymptomatic effects,
- a basic need for chemical hygiene, comparable to the microbiological hygiene which has been cultivated in industrialised societies for more than a century.

## 1. Introduction

Flanders, the northern part of Belgium (Figure 28), is a small (13,413 square kilometres) densely populated area (5.9 million people). It is a heavily industrialised area with many chemical industries, a big steel-producing factory and huge car-assembling factories, along with dense traffic, including intense road transport of goods and intense commuter traffic. Flanders has four hundred and forty-two motor vehicles per thousand inhabitants. Generation of industrial waste amounts to 7.1 million tonnes per year, and generation of municipal waste to 2.6 million tonnes.

From the early 70s on, more and more municipal waste was incinerated. During the early years of incineration, purification of the resulting emissions was limited or even non-existent. Emissions from waste incinerators include, amongst others, carbon monoxide, nitrogen oxides, dust, polycyclic aromatic hydrocarbons, heavy metals, and dioxins. It is, however, with regard to dioxins that the relative contribution of waste incinerators has been most important, as incineration of waste was calculated to be responsible for 59.31 per cent of dioxin emissions in Flanders in 1990. In 1992, dioxin concentrations in the air in Flanders were measured in six locations and varied between 100 and 255 fg TEQ/$m^3$ (Cornelis *et al.*, 1998). Dioxin deposits were measured from 1993 onward at several locations and varied between 0.26 ng TEQ/$m^2$/y (in the city of Mol, 1997) and 374 ng TEQ/$m^2$/y (in the city of Menen, 1993) (Cornelis *et al.*, 1998). Calculations concerning dioxin deposit from 1980 to 1996 due to incineration of municipal waste showed that the area around Wilrijk was amongst the regions that received the highest amounts of dioxins.

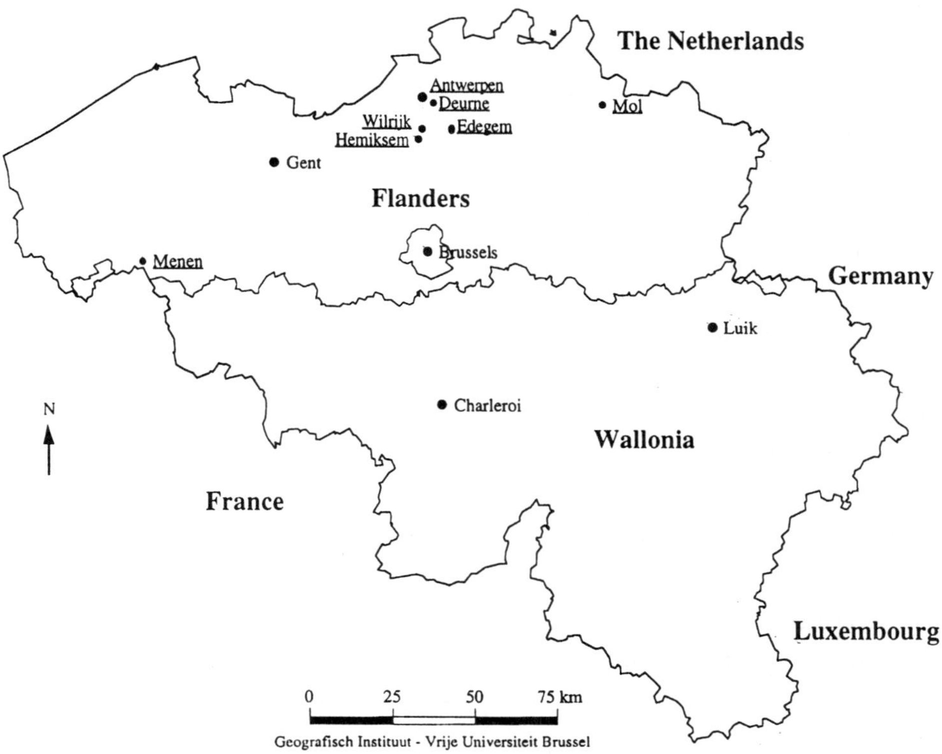


*Figure 28.* Map of Belgium.

A cluster of congenital anomalies was discovered amongst inhabitants of the Neerland neighbourhood in Wilrijk. This neighbourhood is situated between the municipal waste incinerators IHK at Edegem (at a distance of about 800 meters) and ISVAG at Wilrijk (at a distance of about 1200 meters). This finding stirred unrest among the inhabitants and in the Flemish population in general. A popular book (Cremers *et al.*, 1997) was even written on this case. A special commission was set up by the minister responsible for the environment and two health studies were ordered by the Flemish Minister of Health. This paper summarises the results of these studies.

## 2. Chromosomal Aberrations

A first study (Verschaeve and Schoeters, 1998), under the direction of Dr. Verschaeve of the 'Vlaams Instituut voor Technologisch Onderzoek' was aimed at detecting genetic effects of exposure to the incinerator's emissions, as these emissions contain genotoxic agents in addition to dioxins. Twenty-four children from Neerland were compared with twenty children from another neighbourhood (Deurne) in the Antwerp region, as to the prevalence of chromosomal aberrations in metaphases of peripheral lymphocytes. Two hundred metaphases were studied per child.

No difference was found (see Tables 28 and 29). A possible flaw in this study stems from the fact that the total exposure of the two studied populations might have been similar, and that negative confounding might have resulted from the fact that the twenty-four children in the Neerland neighbourhood had six smoking parents, whereas the twenty children in the control group had seventeen smoking parents. Furthermore, it is to be noted that this study was not designed to detect health effects of dioxins, as dioxins have no direct genotoxic activity. Although this study was carefully conducted by experienced researchers, and although the number of subjects included is sufficient in comparison to most other studies intended to detect the genetic effects of exposure to genotoxic agents, its sensitivity is limited. In statistical terms, it probably has the power to exclude an increase in chromosome aberrations of the order of magnitude of a doubling, with more than 95 per cent confidence. However, a doubling in the prevalence of chromosome aberrations in peripheral lymphocytes could correspond to a quite important increase in congenital anomalies, and, in terms of somatic mutations, to a huge increase in the risk of cancer if the doubling was to persist throughout life (van Delft *et al.*, 1998). As we are looking at differences resulting from exposures extending over very long periods, an increase of a few percent in chromosome aberrations could result in, and correspond with, a meaningful health risk.

*Table 28.* Number of cells from children living in the Neerland neighbourhood with chromatid or chromosome aberrations (after Verschaeve and Schoeters, 1998).

| Child # | Number of cells with chromatid type aberrations | Number of cells with chromosome type aberrations |
|---|---|---|
| 1 | 0 | 0 |
| 2 | 0 | 0 |
| 3 | 1 | 0 |
| 4 | 0 | 2 |
| 5 | 2 | 3 |
| 6 | 1 | 2 |
| 7 | 2 | 0 |
| 8 | 0 | 1 |
| 9 | 2 | 3 |
| 10 | 2 | 0 |
| 11 | 0 | 0 |
| 12 | 0 | 0 |
| 13 | 1 | 0 |
| 14 | 0 | 3 |
| 15 | 1 | 1 |
| 16 | 1 | 1 |
| 17 | 0 | 1 |
| 18 | 0 | 1 |
| 19 | 3 | 1 |
| 20 | 0 | 0 |
| 21 | 4 | 1 |
| 22 | 2 | 0 |
| 23 | 2 | 2 |
| 24 | 0 | 2 |
| Sum for all children | 24 | 24 |
| % of cells with aberrations for all children in each group | 0.5 | 0.5 |

*Table 29.* Number of cells from children living in the control area (Deurne) with chromatid or chromosome aberrations (after Verschaeve and Schoeters, 1998).

| Child # | Number of cells with chromatid type aberrations | Number of cells with chromosome type aberrations |
|---|---|---|
| 1 | 0 | 0 |
| 2 | 1 | 0 |
| 3 | 1 | 0 |
| 4 | 2 | 0 |
| 5 | 2 | 0 |
| 6 | 1 | 1 |
| 7 | 1 | 0 |
| 8 | 0 | 0 |
| 9 | 0 | 0 |
| 10 | 3 | 1 |
| 11 | 0 | 0 |
| 12 | 1 | 1 |
| 13 | 1 | 2 |
| 14 | 2 | 0 |
| 15 | 1 | 0 |
| 16 | 2 | 0 |
| 17 | 2 | 3 |
| 18 | 3 | 2 |
| 19 | 3 | 0 |
| 20 | 2 | 0 |
| Sum for all children | 28 | 10 |
| % of cells with aberrations for all children in each group | 0.7 | 0.25 |

## 3. Perinatal Health

A second study, by Aelvoet *et al.* (1998), concerned health problems of children from the Neerland neighbourhood. This study found no difference between the whole of Flanders and the Neerland neighbourhood as to perinatal death. There was, however, a statistically non-significant difference in the incidence of congenital malformations, with an odds ratio of 1.26 (0.80-1.99) (see Table 30). So, for women in the Neerland neighbourhood the likelihood of having a baby with a congenital malformation appears to be 1.26 times greater than for Flemish women in general, with the 95 per cent confidence limits at 0.80 and 1.99 times.

*Table 30.* Incidence of congenital malformations in the Neerland neighbourhood, situated in the vicinity of a household waste incinerator and Flanders (Vlaanderen) as a whole (after Aelvoet *et al.*, 1998).

| **Malformations** | **Place of residence of the mother** | | **Total** |
|---|---|---|---|
| | **Neerland** | **Vlaanderen** | |
| Present | 13 (2.04%) | 8,259 (1.63%) | 8,272 |
| Absent | 623 (97.96%) | 497,737 (98.37%) | 498,360 |
| Total | 636 | 505,996 | 506,632 |

There was also a statistically significant increase in the number of multiple pregnancies, with an odds ratio of 2.6 (2.1-3.3). So for women in the Neerland neighbourhood, the likelihood of having a multiple pregnancy appears to be 2.6 times greater than for Flemish women in general, with the 95 per cent confidence limits at 2.1 and 3.3 times.

*Table 31.* Incidence of multiple pregnancies in mothers living near a household waste incinerator (Neerland neighbourhood) as compared to the incidence in Flanders (Vlaanderen) as a whole (after Aelvoet *et al.*, 1998).

| **Multiple pregnancy** | **Place of residence of the mother** | | **Total** |
|---|---|---|---|
| | **Neerland** | **Vlaanderen** | |
| Present | 55 (8.65%) | 17,601 (3.48%) | 17,656 |
| Absent | 581 (91.35%) | 488,395 (96.52%) | 488,976 |
| Total | 636 | 505,996 | 506,632 |

Parity, age of the mother, sex ratio, neonatal weight and duration of pregnancy were very similar in Neerland and in the whole of Flanders. However, the frequency of medical intervention in the conception was different. For multiple pregnancies, medical intervention occurred in 59 per cent of cases in Neerland, and only in 33.3 per cent in Flanders. The occurrence of medical intervention in single pregnancies showed a similar ratio between Neerland and Flanders as a whole, but at a level that was ten times lower, 5.61 per cent in Neerland against 3.37 in Flanders.

Pregnancies of mothers from the Neerland neighbourhood were also compared with pregnancies of mothers who delivered in the same clinics but who resided elsewhere. Again a statistically non-significant increase in congenital malformations was found; the odds ratio was 1.34 (0.83-2.17) (see tables). For women from the Neerland neighbourhood the likelihood of having a baby with a congenital malformation appears to be 1.34 times greater than for mothers who delivered in the same clinics but who resided elsewhere, with the 95 per cent confidence limits at 0.83 and 2.17 times.

*Table 32.* Comparison of incidence of congenital malformations in mothers living near a household waste incinerator (Neerland neighbourhood) and mothers delivering in the same hospital, but residing elsewhere (other) (after Aelvoet *et al.*, 1998).

| **Malformations** | **Place of residence of the mother** | | **Total** |
|---|---|---|---|
| | **Neerland** | **Other** | |
| Present | 12 (2.08%) | 1,297 (1.56%) | 1,309 |
| Absent | 566 (97.92%) | 82,177 (98.44%) | 82,743 |
| Total | 578 | 83,474 | 84,052 |

After correction for age, sex and multiple pregnancies, the odds ratio for congenital malformations amounted to 1.29 for Neerland mothers, compared to mothers who delivered in the same clinics but who resided elsewhere.

The authors controlled also the relation between duration of residence of the mother or father and occurrence of congenital malformations. The results showed that the increase in relative risk for congenital malformations appeared to be confined to children born from parents who had not resided for a long time in Neerland.

Relation between duration of residence of mother or father and occurrence of multiple pregnancies: duration of exposure (residence) of the mother was not statistically significantly related to occurrence of multiple pregnancies.

## 4. Performance and Health at School Age

In this second study (Aelvoet *et al.*, 1998) the performance at school of children from the Neerland neighbourhood was compared to that of other children from Wilrijk and to the performance of Flemish children in general. Occurrence of failure at school was not increased in Neerland, and there were significantly less children from the Neerland neighbourhood in special education classes.

Moreover, the health status of children from the school in the Neerland neighbourhood was compared to that of a nearby school in Hemiksem. Data concerning the health status were obtained from the School Medical Control files on individual children. The files contain anamnestic lists with data provided by the parents, and data provided by the school physician on the occasion of a medical examination. Anamnestic data include data on pregnancy and birth, first years of life, previous diseases, medical interventions, accidents, medical treatments and the present state of health. Data stemming from the medical examination include further treatment and data concerning referral to other health services.

*Table 33.* Incidence of allergies, common colds and health complaints in children of the third class schools (5 years) living near a household waste incinerator (Neerland neighbourhood) and children living near a metallurgic plant (Hemiksem) (after Aelvoet *et al.*, 1998).

| Pathology or complaint | Cases in Neerland | % in Neerland | Cases in Hemiksem | % in Hemiksem | Fisher's exact test |
|---|---|---|---|---|---|
| Allergy | 10 | 7.2 | 4 | 2.1 | 0.025 |
| Repeated episodes of common cold | 23 | 16.5 | 8 | 4.2 | 0.00017 |
| Health complaints | 40 | 28.8 | 28 | 14.8 | 0.002 |

For the first class of maternal school no significant differences were observed. For the third class of maternal school significant differences were found. Allergies and repeated episodes of the common cold were more frequent in children from Neerland than in children from Hemiksem. Also health problems (complaints) in general were more frequent in Neerland than in Hemiksem.

*Table 34.* Use of medication and incidence of allergies in children of the third class of primary school (9 years) living near a household waste incinerator (Neerland neighbourhood) and living near a metallurgic plant (Hemiksem) (after Aelvoet *et al.*, 1998).

| | **Cases in Neerland** | **% in Neerland** | **Cases in Hemiksem** | **% in Hemiksem** | **Fisher's exact test** |
|---|---|---|---|---|---|
| Used medication since last visit | 10 | 11.0 | 3 | 2.5 | 0.012 |
| Allergy | 10 | 11 | 5 | 4.2 | 0.051 |

For the third class of primary school significant differences were found concerning the prevalence of allergies and the occurrence of 'use of medication' since the last examination by the school health service. Use of medication can be considered an indirect measure of ill health caused by pollution.

## 5. Discussion

Do these data imply that these studies provide a fair idea of the impact of these waste incinerators on the health of the population concerned? No, for the following reasons:

- if somatic (and possibly germ line) genetic effects are present, they can be expected to be of low intensity, below the level of sensitivity of the present observations. Such genetic effects could still have a significant health impact;
- epidemiological data are only available concerning a few pathologic conditions. Conceivably, a more detailed in-depth analysis of the health status of children from the Neerland neighbourhood might reveal other health effects possibly related to pollution;

- data on internal doses (especially concerning dioxins) are lacking. Blood levels of dioxin-like substances, and especially the monitoring of dioxin-like substances in umbilical cord blood would provide a much firmer basis for assessing exposure and for linking possible health effects with exposure;
- data on early (pre-symptomatic) biological effects other than chromosomal aberrations are lacking;
- comparing two populations who reside at different distances from an incinerator does not permit an assessment of the true, total impact of incineration on human health, as incinerators are not the only important sources of pollution in the region and as exposure to dioxin-like substances (and possibly also to other air pollutants) is mainly through food. Moreover, Hemiksem, which also has industrial plants, is an unfortunate choice for a control region, as some data concerning dioxin deposition suggest that Hemiksem might have the same level of pollution by dioxins as the Neerland neighbourhood.

This ASPIS workshop aims at contributing to the raising of awareness of the effects of environmental pollution on health. Therefore, it is important to raise the issue of physical-chemical hygiene. Physical-chemical hygiene consists of limiting, as much as possible, exposure to biologically active radiation, reactive chemical substances, and receptor-binding, hormone-disrupting chemical substances.

About a hundred years ago the introduction of anti-microbial hygiene allowed us to reduce the incidence of and mortality from infectious diseases. Now, if we want to reduce the incidence of and mortality from cancer, and probably also from other 'diseases of civilisation', (along with infertility and congenital anomalies), we need to introduce physical-chemical hygiene. Why is this so?

1. Epidemiology proves that cancer is due, in at least 80 per cent of cases, to external factors. The incidence of cancer has risen considerably in the developed regions of the world (Davis *et al.*, 1994; Adami *et al.*, 1993).
2. Both epidemiological and experimental evidence points to an important role of mutations in the process of carcinogenesis (Van Larebeke, 1997).

3. DNA damage by endogenous agents is often repaired more quickly and more efficiently than damage by recently introduced exogenous chemical agents (Deman and Van Larebeke, 1997).
4. Co-carcinogenic and synergistic interactions are probably very important in causing cancer in humans.
5. There are very many carcinogens (probably some 10 per cent of chemicals have some carcinogenic potency) (Huff and Hoel, 1992; Huff, 1993).
6. The great majority of carcinogens present in our environment have not been identified.
7. Epigenetic carcinogens, such as hormone-like substances, act at very low doses.
8. Choosing priorities is hampered by huge uncertainties in comparative risk assessment (Finkel, 1995).

Besides the need for chemical hygiene, another implication of the above is that measuring chemical substances in the environment or even measuring internal doses is not sufficient. Biological tests must be used in an integrated way to detect pre-symptomatic biological effects of pollution, and to detect them as early as possible and with the best sensitivity.

## References

Adami, H.O., Bergstrom, R., Sparen, P., and Baron, J. (1993) Increasing cancer risk in younger birth cohorts in Sweden, *Lancet* **I 341 (8848)**, 773-777.

Aelvoet, W., Nelen, V., Schoeters, G., Vanoverloop, J., Wallijn, E. and Vlietinck, R. (1998) Risico op gezondheidsschade bij kinderen van de Neerlandwijk te Wilrijk, Studie uitgevoerd in opdracht van de Vlaamse Minister bevoegd voor het Gezondheidsbeleid, Document 1998/TOX/R/030. (in Dutch)

Cornelis, C., De Fré, R., Nouwen, J., and Schoeters, G. (1998) Voorstel van normen voor dioxines in lucht en depositie, VITO report 1998/DIA/R20, opgesteld in opdracht van de Vlaamse Milieumaatschappij, Erembodegem, Belgium. (in Dutch)

Cremers, P., Van Laerhoven, B. and Willems, R. (1997) Moorddadig milieu in Vlaanderen. Moeder waarom leven wij? Icarus, Standaard Uitgeverij, Antwerpen, Belgium. (in Dutch)

Davis, D.L., Dinse, G.E., and Hoel, D.G. (1994) Decreasing cardiovascular disease and increasing cancer among whites in the United States from 1973 through 1987. Good news and bad news, *JAMA* **271** **(6)**, 431-437.

Deman, J., and Van Larebeke, N. (1997) Beschadiging en herstel van DNA. Ontstaan van mutaties, Rapport aan de Vlaamse Milieumaatschappij. (in Dutch)

Finkel, A.M. (1995) Toward less misleading comparisons of uncertain risks: the example of aflatoxin and alar, *Environ. Health Perspect.* **103** **(4)**, 376-385.

Huff, J. (1993) Issues and controversies surrounding qualitative strategies for identifying and forecasting cancer causing agents in the human environment, *Pharmacol. Toxicol.* **72** **(Suppl 1)**, 12-27.

Huff, J., and Hoel, D. (1992) Perspective and overview of the concepts and value of hazard identification as the initial phase of risk assessment for cancer and human health, *Scand. J. Work. Environ. Health* **18** **(Suppl 1)**, 83-89.

Schoeters, G., Cornelis, C., De Fré, R., Hooghe, R., Colier, M., Maes, A., Mensinck, C., Nouwen, J., Patyn, J., Verschaeve, L., Viaene, P., and Geuzens, P. (1998) Studie van gezondheidsaspecten en gezondheidsrisico's tengevolge van de milieuverontreiniging in de Neerlandwijk te Wilrijk, VITO report 1998/ TOX/R/009, Mol, Belgium. (in Dutch)

van Delft, J.H., Baan, R.A., and Roza, L. (1998) Biological effect markers for exposure to carcinogenic compound and their relevance for risk assessment, *Crit. Rev. Toxicol.* **28** **(5)**, 477-510.

Van Larebeke, N. (1997) *Invloed van het leefmilieu en van de vervuiling ervan op de kankerincidentie. Gegevens en inzichten die wijzen op het belang van milieufactoren in het ontstaan van kanker bij de mens en op de noodzaak van het invoeren van een fysisch-chemische hygiëne*, Vlaamse Milieumaatschappij, Erembodegem, Belgium. (in Dutch)

Verschaeve, L. and Schoeters, G. (1998) Cytogenetisch populatieonderzoek: commentaren bij het cytogenetisch onderzoek van kinderen in de Neerlandwijk, VITO report 1998/R/TOX/045, Mol, Belgium. (in Dutch)

# IMPACTS OF INADEQUATE OR NEGLIGENT WASTE DISPOSAL ON WILDLIFE AND DOMESTIC ANIMALS: RELEVANCE FOR HUMAN HEALTH

G. STAATS DE YANES[1]
C.V. HOWARD[2]
[1]*WHO-Centre*
*Tierärztlichen Hochschule Hannover*
*Bünteweg 2*
*D-30559 Hannover*
*GERMANY*
[2]*University of Liverpool*
*Fetal & Infant Toxico-Pathology*
*P.O. Box 147*
*L69 7ZA Liverpool*
*UNITED KINGDOM*

**Summary**

Humans are at the top of the food web, and are therefore particularly vulnerable to exposure to those pollutants that are persistent and which bioconcentrate. The major route of human intake of these compounds is food of animal origin. Release and cycling of these compounds in the human food chain is an important problem.

Therefore this chapter is intended to give insight into the complex issue of 'waste as a source for environmental contaminants', with particular emphasis on the accumulation and effects of environmental contaminants on wildlife and domestic animals and the



*P. Nicolopoulou-Stamati et al. (eds.), Health Impacts of Waste Management Policies,* 251–281.

relevance for human health. Examples and studies related to the release of toxic substances into the environment are reported and accordingly waste sources and types are classified. Additionally a list of substances involved is provided, which represent examples of relevant groups of pollutants.

Monitoring the health status and contamination of a wildlife population can be an important tool in early warning systems, in order to protect human health. Effects on wildlife populations, if observed, can point to environmental problems long before effects in humans might be observed. Animal species can be used as indicators for pollution.

Waste management and its effects on human health are global problems. This is because of factors such as: global distillation of compounds, the global trade of animal feed, animal products, waste (legal or illegal) and, last but not least, global tourism. Therefore this is a problem that cannot be solved solely on a national basis but only by an international co-operation in identifying sources, decreasing or stopping emissions and developing strategies to avoid the intake of hazardous amounts of contaminants.

In conclusion, strategies for the avoidance of the release into the environment are discussed. Recent developments in the contamination of animal feeds in Europe, which have been widely spread throughout the food distribution system, act to highlight the unfortunate consequences that can arise from using the food chain as a sink for industrial waste.

## 1. Introduction

Previous papers in this volume have mainly dealt with waste landfilling and incineration and the related environmental contaminant dioxin. This paper introduces further aspects and types of waste into the discussion. We define waste in this context to include all material that has to be disposed of

⇒ because it has fulfilled its use and lost its value in a former application, e.g. lime;

⇒ because it is an unwanted by-product, such as sewage, carcasses, etc.;

⇒ because it occupies room that is otherwise required, such as sediments in harbours or navigable rivers.

In the first section we give as comprehensive a list as possible of waste types and contaminants involved in addition to those associated with incineration and dioxins. This is illustrated by examples of substances released in association with certain waste disposal methods.

The second and the third part then focus jointly on persistent organic pollutants. The second part deals specifically with the global distribution of these compounds, while the third section 'Health Effects and Contamination in Animals and Relevance for Human Health' addresses the following points and their relevance for human health:

- relating to wildlife, abundance and health effects are discussed with consideration of diseases/epidemics, decline and extinction. As a consequence we examine the implications for necessary research into effects on humans. Furthermore the identification of indicator species and monitoring are mentioned;
- with respect to domestic animals we consider health effects, human environment sharing, food of animal origin and the impact of feed stuffs on human health.

In the conclusion we discuss possible strategies for the reduction and avoidance of the introduction of persistent hazardous substances into the food chain.

## 2. Examples of Problematic Hazardous Substances and Related Waste Types

In the following section, some cases of environmental contamination are described, in which waste management has failed to protect the environment, either because no or insufficient regulation is currently in place (e.g. insufficient research had been carried out previously to justify regulation or no agreements could be achieved), regulation has not been implemented properly or controls are not sufficient. A good example of insufficient management to avoid further contamination is given in Box 1 for PCBs.

*Box 1.* A short history of PCBs.

| | |
|---|---|
| 1881 | first synthesised |
| Since 1929 | industrial production |
| 1966 | PCBs found in Baltic wildlife |
| 1970 | use in 'open' systems banned |
| Until 1990 | production stopped in most OECD countries |
| | banned in all applications in some countries |
| 1998 | still in use in closed systems (transformers, capacitors) |
| | still produced in e.g. Russia (Int. Environ. Rep., 1998) |
| End of 1999 | deadline for phase-out agreed on by the Ministerial Conference of the North Sea EC States in 1990 |
| 2010 | deadline for phase-out under the 1996 EC Directive on PCB disposal |

- i.e. **33 years** after the initial knowledge about persistence, atmospheric transport and bio-accumulation, there is still no world-wide ban on the production and use of PCBs.
- The estimated total production of PCB in OECD countries was 1.5 million tons (Bletchly, 1984).
- Estimation of distribution of PCB might differ (see e.g. Marquenie and Reijnders, 1989; Tanabe, 1988); most estimates in the literature are closer to the latter reference:
  - ≈ 2/3 still in use (mainly closed systems) or deposited in landfills and dumps
  - ≈ 1/3 has reached the environment, of which
    - ≈ 2/3 reached open oceans (considered as final sink) and
    - ≈ 1/3 remains in terrestrial/coastal areas (water, sediments, soil, biota)
  - ≈ 4% has been destroyed

The following examples of inadequate waste management help explain why contamination levels can increase both locally and/or globally, or no further decrease of levels of pollutants can be achieved despite the implementation of regulations reducing new releases. Although at first sight, these incidents might appear disconnected and unrelated, there is a common theme which centres on the legal or illegal disposal of persistent pollutants, some of which can pose a threat through the animal side of the food chain.

- Sediments dredged from rivers and harbours have been dumped in coastal waters (near a conservation area) and onto grazing land (this is general practice). These sediments have been highly contaminated with several compounds. Especially high concentrations of organo-tins were determined (up to 90,000 μg TBT/kg dry matter) (Gülden *et al.*, 1997). These compounds are of special concern at the moment. They are known to cause, at very low levels (3 ng/l), pseudohermaphroditism, known as imposex, in female dogwhelk snails resulting in sterility (Reijnders and Brasseur, 1992). There is no international, and at best only regional, regulation of maximum concentrations for dumping these sludges. There is some evidence for toxicity in humans as well. Such sludges ending up on grazing land are likely to find their way into the human food chain, via animals.

- Hexachlorobenzene (HCB) was formerly used as a fungicide, but has now been phased out because of its toxicity. Since then the main source has become industrial waste; e.g. dumping at sea has been the sole source of HCB in the North Sea. The Dioxin'98 Conference heard reports of increasing concentrations of HCB in humans, near industrial sites in Spain (Ozalla *et al.*, 1998). Only recently, van Birgelen (1998) reported the dioxin-like toxicity of HCB and that, in some countries, such as Spain, Slovakia and the Czech Republic, HCB might contribute up to a factor of 6 to the total dioxin-like toxicity (TEQ) in breast milk. That showed that even with well-known toxic organochlorines, the most routinely available toxicity testing wasn't performed, despite the widespread use of this chemical in industry.

- Crematoria are sources for the emission of high levels of dioxins (e.g. Cuijpers *et al.*, 1998).

- Drugs and partially degraded drugs (antibiotics, hormones, blood-lipid-level regulating drugs, analgesics, antiseptics, beta-blockers, anti-epileptic drugs, etc.) have been found in sewage, treated water, streams, rivers, lakes and drinking water (ENS, 1998). Little is known about the eco-toxicology of drugs (DFG, 1997). Only recently has eco-toxicological testing started for newly developed substances and been discussed for old drugs. Test systems are under development. In areas of industrialised livestock production, drugs and their metabolites might be of special relevance.

- Antibiotics and their metabolites can be found in high concentrations in animal excreta, which might have an influence on bacterial selection with antibiotic resistance genes (DFG, 1997).

- Natural and synthetic hormones, chemicals with endocrine activity, have been detected at bioactive levels (e.g. causing increased vitellogenin production, gonadal changes) downstream from sewage plants (Purdom *et al.*, 1994).

- Since 1984, the Greek steel company Larco has been dumping toxic sludges containing heavy metals into the Gulf of Evoikos near Euböa. This contravenes international law and the Greek government knows about it, according to Greenpeace, but has taken no action (Greenpeace, 1999).

- In the middle of Hannover, Germany, beside a very busy road, a hundred condensers containing PCBs were dumped (HAZ, 1998).

Hazardous substance-classes that are involved include:

- heavy metals;
- additives in plastics such as phthalates or bisphenol-A, which are known for their endocrine disrupting activities;
- organo-tins;
- pharmaceuticals (hormones, antibiotics, etc.);
- persistent organohalogens.

The next two sections of this chapter will focus on organohalogen compounds. This is not to ignore the fact that there are many other hazardous substances that are or might be of a similar relevance in this context.

Persistent organohalogens can be roughly separated into three groups (Table 35).

*Table 35.* Groups of persistent organohalogens.

| a. Industrial chemicals | b. Pesticides | c. Contaminants |
|---|---|---|
| polychlorinated biphenyls (PCB) | DDT | polychlorinated dibenzodioxins (PCDD) |
| polybrominated biphenyls (PBB) | toxaphenes | polychlorinated dibenzofurans (PCDF) |
| hexachlorobenzene (HCB) | lindane | polybrominated and mixed PxDF/D* |
| polybrominated diphenyl ethers (PBDE) | etc. | etc. |
| tetrabrombisphenol-A | | |
| etc. | | |

* (UBA, 1989)

### *a. Industrial Chemicals*

Due to their properties of thermal, chemical (resistance to bases, acids, oxidation, hydrolysis) and electrical stability, low flammability, low vapour pressure, low water solubility and high lipophilicity, industrial chemicals are used in a long list of applications, either pure or as additives. Examples include flame retardants, oils, fluids in hydraulic systems, transformers, capacitors, plasticisers, lubricants, paints, solvents, waxes, agents for sealing, lamination, impregnation, pesticides, cement, plaster.

Detailed information about production, properties, applications, contaminated products and sources for environmental contamination can be found in Kimbrough and Jensen (1989).

### *b. Pesticides*

Organochlorine pesticides were developed because of their relatively low acute toxicity to humans, their stability and therefore long-term effect. They were produced to be released directly into the environment. Their persistence in the environment, bio-accumulation and bioconcentration and long-term low-dose toxicity were not considered at that time. The ongoing use of some of them in some applications is strongly to be questioned, because of their known negative effects.

### c. *Contaminants*

These compounds have never been produced intentionally. Halogenated products, such as the above-mentioned pesticides or chemicals, can contain considerable amounts of these unwanted contaminants. Other sources come from low temperature burning, accidental fires, or heating and use of halogenated compounds.

*Box 2.* Waste types as sources of persistent organic pollutants.

- incinerators (municipal, hazardous, industrial waste)
  * fugitive gases
  * fly ash
  * bottom ash
- industrial emissions (steel, paper, chemical industry)
  * fugitive gases
  * wastewater
- human excreta
- sewage plants
  * sludge
  * wastewater
- landfill dumping sites
- waste disposal
  * hazardous/non-hazardous
- dumping and incineration at sea
- tanker cleaning offshore
- animal excreta
- crematoria
- export of waste/hazardous waste
- selling or transferring of old technologies to developing countries, and/or countries with less strict legislation, might be considered as a special form of waste management.

The Swedish EPA (1998) published a very comprehensive report on persistent organic pollutants and the related problems.

In Box 2 a variety of **waste types** is listed that might be involved as sources of environmental and health problems.

## 3. Global Distillation of Persistent Organic Pollutants

Once persistent pollutants are released into the environment, for many, virtually no degradation takes place, because of their stability. However they don't remain stationary. A partitioning process between surrounding matrices takes place (Tanabe *et al.*, 1994).

### *3.1. Volatilisation*

Persistent compounds pass into the air from contaminated terrestrial and coastal surfaces in industrialised areas or near the sites of application. This process is enhanced by higher temperatures, such as occur in warm regions.

### *3.2. Atmospheric Transport*

The compounds are transported on air currents, from highly polluted areas to lower contaminated areas, such as e.g. open oceans, where re-solution at the surface takes place. Due to these processes, these compounds can be found all over the world, not only near the places where they were originally used.

These processes lead to the current findings of

- decreasing concentrations in industrial countries and coastal areas, after the implementation of restrictions in use, and phase-out, of persistent substances,
- relatively high concentrations in remote or previously pristine areas, such as open oceans or non-coastal sediments. Trends are not unequivocal in either direction.

### *3.3. Cold Condensation*

Concern about the polar regions is increasing. Due to global distillation and cold condensation, environmental pollutants have reached high concentrations in these sensitive ecosystems (e.g. AMAP, 1998; Kidd *et al.*, 1995). As a consequence of the recent findings of cold condensation at high altitudes in the Canadian Rocky Mountains (Blais *et al.*, 1998), research in the near future might focus on wildlife and populations in similar areas, such as Andean areas in South America. People there are living above 4000 m and grazing their alpacas at up to more than 6000 m. The polar ecosystems and mountainous areas must be carefully monitored for effects.

## 4. Health Effects and Contamination in Animals and the Relevance of these for Human Health

### 4.1. *Wildlife*

#### 4.1.1. *Abundance and health effects*

There are reviews on effects that have been monitored in wildlife populations, such as declines in population size, regional extinction, outbreaks of epizootic diseases, increased mortality and reproductive failures. These were considered to be due or partly due to exposure to organohalogen compounds (e.g. in Gilbertson, 1989; Reijnders and Brasseur, 1992).

Here, briefly, are some of these effects:

- *series of morbilli virus outbreaks in recent years*

  1987/8 bottlenose dolphin, East Coast, USA (Duignan *et al.*, 1996)
  1988/9 common seal, North Sea (Heide-Jørgensen *et al.*, 1992)
  1989 Baikal seals, Lake Baikal (Grachev *et al.*, 1989)
  1990/1 striped dolphins, Mediterranean Sea (Aguilar and Borrell, 1994)
  1997 monk seals, Mediterranean Sea (Harwood, 1998; Hernandez *et al.*, 1998)

  In nearly all these cases, algal toxins and environmental contaminants have been discussed as aetiologic agents, in addition to organochlorines. At least in the seal epidemics in the North Sea (Heide-Jørgensen *et al.*, 1992; Simmonds *et al.*, 1993) and in the dolphin epidemic in the Mediterranean Sea (Kannan *et al.*, 1993; Aguilar and Borrell, 1994), the influence of contamination with organochlorine compounds on mortality was evident. In Baikal seals, PCB and PCDD/F concentrations are similar to those found in other highly contaminated areas such as the Baltic Sea.

- *disease complex in Baltic seals*
  In Baltic seals, a disease complex was described (Bergman and Olsson, 1985) and was compared with Cushing's disease. Symptoms were uterine stenoses and occlusions, adrenocortical hyperplasia, alterations in skin and claws, intestine and kidneys, and deformation of the skeleton. Helle (1981) reported that uterus occlusions occurred in 50 per cent of the ringed seals. The adrenal toxicity of DDT metabolites may be involved (Lund, 1994).
  A collection of skulls of seals revealed, from the 1950's onwards, a rising incidence of deformations of jaw bones, due to ulcers in the mouth, in up to 50 per cent of the population (Swedish EPA, 1998). Organochlorine contamination of the Baltic Sea is the most obvious reason.

- *frogs with malformations and extinction of frog species world-wide*
  The causes of the phenomenon are still not fully understood, but seem to be partly due to application of pesticides on agricultural land (Montague, 1998).

- *health problems and reproductive failure in Beluga whales, St-Lawrence Estuary, USA*
  Beluga whales in the St-Lawrence Estuary, which is highly contaminated with organochlorine compounds, suffer reproductive disorders, have a high cancer rate and adrenocortical alterations (Gilbertson, 1989; DeGuise *et al.*, 1995; Heide-Jørgensen and Reeves, 1996; Lair *et al.*, 1997).

- *hermaphroditic polar bears in Spitzbergen*
  The increasing incidence of hermaphroditic polar bears in Spitzbergen was probably caused by high levels of PCBs, which were released by a coal-mine in that area (Wiig *et al.*, 1998).

From the literature, as well as from this short list, the following conclusions can be drawn:

***Species at risk***

- have a high position in the aquatic food web
    * piscivorous birds (e.g. gulls, terns, cormorants, eagles)
    * piscivorous terrestrial mammals (e.g. mink, otter)
    * marine mammals (e.g. seals, dolphins, whales)

For example, toothed marine mammals have generally higher concentrations of persistent organic pollutants than non-toothed. That is due to the fact that the former mainly feed on fish while the latter feed on organisms lower down the aquatic food web. The levels of pollutants such as PCBs in top predators have been shown to be elevated several million-fold compared with the surrounding water (biomagnification). Top predators in the terrestrial food chain, like foxes or dogs, have a much higher and different metabolic activity towards these compounds and therefore don't bio-accumulate them to the same extent as marine mammals (Tanabe, 1988).

***Species at special risk***

- have a top position in the aquatic food web
    * polar bears
    * killer whales

These have marine mammals in their diet and are consequently one further step up the food chain than fish-eating animals.

*4.1.2. Implications for necessary research into effects on humans*

Table 36 lists examples of research pointing to the issues of how findings in animals serve to illustrate the need to intensify the evaluation of effects on wildlife populations, in order to learn about impacts on human health.

*Table 36.* Relationship between findings in animals and impacts on humans.

| Wildlife findings | Research in humans |
|---|---|
| Discovery of PCB in wildlife | determination of levels in humans |
| Reproductive failure in wildlife | - monitoring of hormone-disrupting substances in humans<br>- epidemiological research on effects in humans<br>- design appropriate animal experiments, to estimate the hazards to humans |
| High susceptibility of piscivorous animals* | epidemiological studies in fishermen and their families in Great Lakes area, Sweden, Farøes Islands (Grandjean *et al.*, 1995) |

* Surprisingly, the research in Inuit Indians was prompted by the search for a 'clean' unexposed control group, not because of high exposure to polar bears and killer whales that feed on seals, which also contribute to the Inuit food supply. Inuits have been revealed to be highly exposed (Dewailly *et al.*, 1994; Ayotte *et al.*, 1995; Ayotte *et al.*, 1996).

Despite the high levels of pollution of some parts of the Mediterranean Sea (Aguilar and Borrell, 1994), apparently no epidemiological study has been performed in exposed populations in this area. A Mediterranean Monitoring Programme including all coastal countries is planned for seafood.

### *4.1.3. Monitoring*

Monitoring can include recording of

- *pathology data* from animals dead or alive, such as uterine occlusions in Baltic seals or occurrence of chickedema disease in fish-eating birds in the Great Lake area (Gilbertson *et al.*, 1991).
- *population data:* for example, otter and eagle populations that declined dramatically with increasing concentrations of organohalogen compounds, especially PCB and DDT, despite the improvement of habitat conditions, are now recovering in several European countries. This indicates that concentrations of the causal agents have been falling (e.g. Swedish EPA, 1998; Mason, 1998).

- *reproductive success*, as offspring per adult (female), is a part of the previous point, but as many of these pollutants have a negative impact on reproduction it is mentioned separately.
- levels of hazardous substances or body burdens in wildlife species.

Monitoring can give information about environmental contamination according to
- time trends as mentioned above with otter and eagle populations in several parts of Europe.
- regional trends as the previously described disease complex occurs in Baltic seals in some areas of the Baltic Sea but not in others nor in the North Sea. Chickedema disease in birds of some areas of the Great Lakes but not in others provides another example.

*Advantages of monitoring substances in wildlife* result from
- *accumulation in the food chain* so that concentrations can be detected more easily than the
- *very low levels in other environmental material* such as air, soil or water. Therefore
- *comparably low sensitivity of analytical methods* is required (cheaper, less time consuming).

  Samples from animals are usually
- *easier to obtain than human material.*
- *Time and regional trends* can be observed more easily, due to
  * *shorter life cycle* compared to humans and to
  * *well-known feeding habits relating to area and available food sources.*

### 4.1.4. *Indicator species*

Characteristics of the chosen species are:
- *high sensitivity* to the contaminant
- *the development of obvious effects* that are therefore easily detectable.

Possible applications are:
- monitor contamination status, time and temporal trends in a habitat, via monitoring the indicator species in its natural habitat;

- expose the indicator species to an environment that needs to be tested for contamination;
- expose this indicator species under experimental conditions to further contaminants that are expected to cause similar toxic effects (screening of substances) or to mixtures of substances to assess their effect.

For example, systems have been developed, which use fish species to monitor oestrogenic substances (e.g. Sumpter and Jobling, 1995; Allen *et al.,* 1999; Harries *et al.*, 1997 and 1999). These have been used for risk assessment of hormonally active substances under laboratory conditions, as well as for detection of oestrogenic substances downstream of sewage plants (e.g. natural oestrogens, ethinylestradiol) and industrial sites (e.g. bisphenol-A).

### *4.2. Domestic Animals*

Health effects in domestic animals may be of relevance for humans, as domestic animals share the same environment, so they may sometimes indicate contamination before effects in humans are obvious. To our knowledge no epidemiological study in pet animals living in the vicinity of an industrial plant has been performed yet. Due to their relative longevity, and to the fact that they have a restricted range, such pets would probably be much more sensitive indicators for a local source of pollution.

With farm animals, the problem is that only acute effects would be detected easily, because farm animals have a relatively short life span. Long-term low-dose toxicity is very unlikely, therefore, to be detected in farm animals. It would, however, be interesting to study the influence of exposure to different levels of organohalogen compounds or other contaminants on performance of livestock in terms of breeding or fattening.

Death or illness of farm animals due to persistent organic pollutants have been reported, related to accidents in a chemical plant, such as in Seveso, where large amounts of dioxins were released into the environment and sheep in the vicinity died, or in the USA, where polybrominated biphenyls have been fed accidentally to farm animals. In Belgium, illegal waste disposal of PCB-transformer oil into animal feed was related to acute and subacute illness (Mengelers *et al.*, 1999), but usually waste is related to increased levels of pollutants in farm animal products. This is the topic of the following paragraphs.

Food is the major route for the intake of lipophilic, bio-accumulating compounds in humans as shown in Table 37 for PCDDs and PCDFs. But the percentage of total intake might be influenced considerably if there are other sources of exposure. That is even indicated by simply comparing the average data of the three different countries. While in Canada non-food exposure is of little importance, it contributes about 7 per cent in the Netherlands. Differences in the application of potentially contaminated chemicals or in building materials at home or at work might play a role.

*Table 37.* Estimated contributions of ambient, food and non-food sources in total daily exposures to PCDDs and PCDFs for the general population of Canada (Birmingham *et al.*, 1989a and b), Germany (Beck *et al.*, 1992) and the Netherlands (Theelen, 1991); (Liem, 1999).

| **Route of exposure** | **Canada** | | **Germany** | | **the Netherlands** | |
|---|---|---|---|---|---|---|
| | (pg/day) | (%) | (pg/day) | (%) | (pg/day) | (%) |
| Air and soil | 5.1 | (3.5) | 4.5 | (3.2) | 3.2 | (2.5) |
| Food | 139.7 | (96.1) | 131.2 | (93.7) | 110.2 | (86.6) |
| Non-food | 0.3 | (0.2) | 5.0 | (3.6) | 9.1 | (7.1) |
| Total | 145 | | 140 | | 127 | |

Food of animal origin is the most important source as shown in Table 38. Levels of dioxins, furans and dioxin-like PCBs in TEQ in fat from different foods in the Netherlands are given. To determine TEQ, the concentrations of the compounds are multiplied by a factor which quantifies their dioxin-like activity relative to 2,3,7,8-tetrachlor-dibenzodioxin. Fish, raw fish oils, game and horse are shown to have comparably high levels. But without data about consumption of a special foodstuff within a population or a subgroup, the relevance of the high levels can't be estimated. For example, game can contribute a high percentage to the dietary intake in the case of keen hunters who consume their game; while in the general population even a relatively high level of contaminants is of minor relevance because game is rarely consumed. Levels of dioxin in milk fat are shown to vary enormously between different samples. In milk itself due to its low fat content, that might not matter too much, in view of the contribution to the dietary intake; but in dairy products with a high content of milk fat, such as cheese or butter, it is highly relevant.

*Table 38.* Range of concentrations of PCDDs, PCDFs and non-ortho PCBs (in pg TEQ/g fat) in selected food groups in industrialised countries as reported by various authors (Liem, 1999).

| Food group | PCDDs and PCDFs (pg TEQ/g fat) | Non-ortho PCBs (pg TEQ/g fat) |
|---|---|---|
| Dairy products | 0.2 - 4.3 | 0.5 - 1.8 |
| Farm milk (a) | 0.6 - 70 | |
| Beef fat | 0.3 - 7.2 | 0.9 & 2.4 |
| Mutton fat | 1.2 - 1.8 | 2.0 |
| Pork fat | 0.2 - 0.6 | 0.2 |
| Chicken/poultry fat | 0.2 - 2.3 | (<) 1.6 |
| Horse fat | 14 | 25 |
| Meat products | 0.6 - 2.5 | 0.5 & 1.3 |
| Nuts | 0.2 | 0.05 |
| Eggs | 0.2 - 2.0 | 0.9 & 1.8 |
| Cereals | 0.3 - 0.4 | 0.2 - 1.2 |
| Lean sea fish | <21 - 49 | 20 - 160 |
| Freshwater fish | 0.8 - 46 | 2.9 - 540 |
| Fatty sea fish | 6.8 - 34 | 11 - 160 |
| Game | 17 | 17 |
| Vegetables | 0.1 (b) | 0.015 - 0.4 (b) |
| Vegetable fats and oils | 0.02 & 0.03 | 0.01 |
| Fish oils (raw) | 0.1 - 80 | 0.5 - 12 |
| Fish oils (refined) | 0.1 - 1.8 | 0.3 - 3.4 |

(a) Milk collected in urban and industrial areas in the period 1990-1993

(b) Levels on wet weight basis.

In Figure 29, in addition to the TEQ levels of dioxins and dioxin-like PCBs in fresh weight of different food sources, information about the corresponding average consumption per person per year is given. Consequently the average daily intake per person in TEQs, related to the food item, is calculated for the Swedish population.

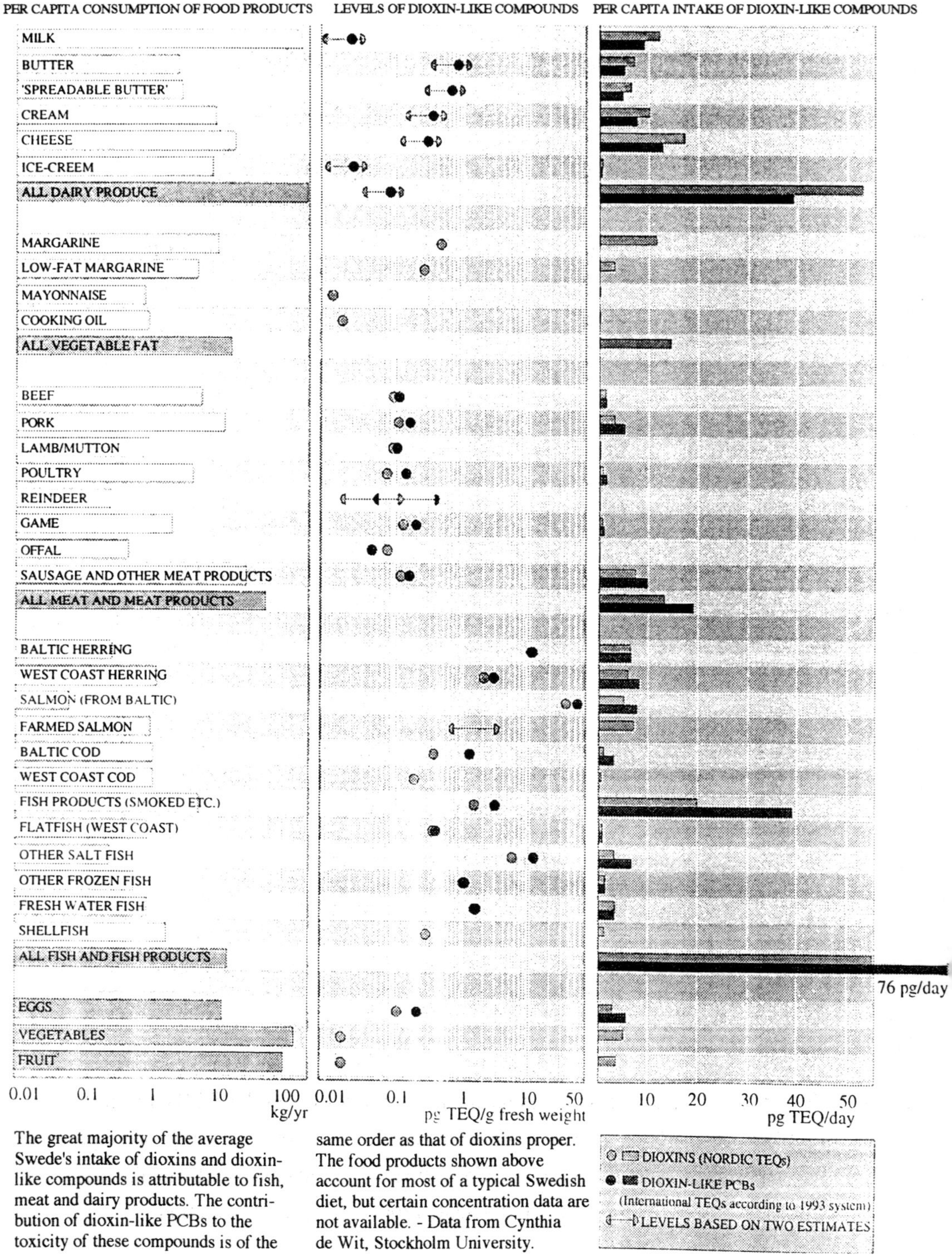


*Figure 29.* Dioxins and dioxin-like PCBs in Swedish food (Swedish EPA, 1998).

Fish and fish products contribute most of the dietary intake; a high contamination level is accompanied by a high consumption of fish and fish products in Sweden. In comparison, milk has very low TEQ levels but is paired with a very high consumption. In consequence, it contributes considerably to the dietary intake.

Figures 30 and 31 show the relative intake of dioxin- and PCB-TEQ via different foods in pre-school children in the Netherlands. This data illustrates the extreme importance of a good control of these compounds in foods of animal origin. Especially for cows' milk, that contributes 50 per cent (PCB) and 43 per cent (dioxin) to the dietary intake. It seems to be extremely important to guarantee levels as low as achievable and this illustrates the need to consider controlling the animal feedstock.

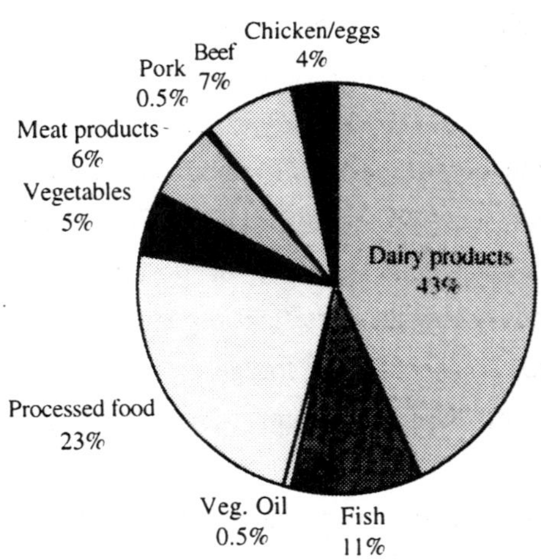


*Figure 30.* Dioxin TEQ in pre-school children in the Netherlands (after Patandin, 1999).

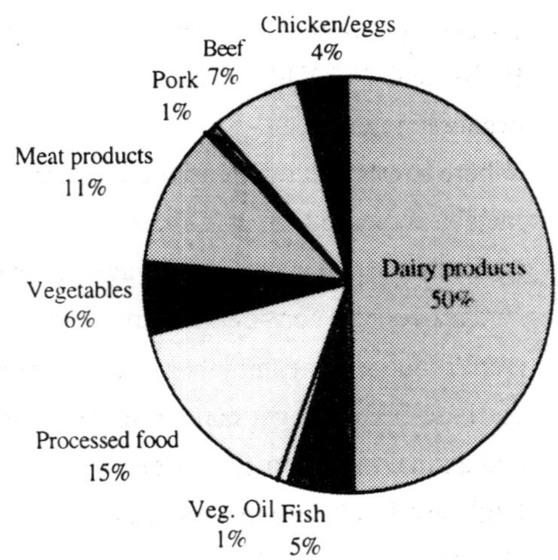


*Figure 31.* Planar PCB-TEQ in pre-school children in the Netherlands (after Patandin, 1999).

Feed is the major route of intake in livestock. Sources of contamination are:

- use of persistent pesticides and pesticides contaminated with persistent organohalogens;
- fish and fish products;
- animals fed on fish products (e.g. slaughterhouse offals);
- incineration sites;
- sewage sludge;

- waste effluents;
- flooding of pastures;
- industrial sites.

In the following section a few examples will be given:

- High concentrations of PCBs and DDT have been detected in fish oils used as dietary supplements for human use (MAFF, 1997c; Stringer *et al.*, 1996; Jacobs and Johnston, 1995). Technology to reduce concentrations in oils is available, but apparently not always applied (Brevik *et al.*, 1990). If this is true for human uses, it will be even more significant for animal uses.
- Farmed trout and salmon are usually fed on diets containing a high percentage of fish or fish products. Depending on toxaphene content in diet, farmed fish exhibited high concentrations of toxaphene (Oetjen and Karl, 1997). The same is the case with PCBs and PCDD/Fs (Isosaari *et al.*, 1998) and probably most other persistent organohalogens.
- Where sewage sludge is applied to farm land, persistent organic pollutants and heavy metals increased in products from cows (ENDS report, 1993; Fries, 1996; McLachlin *et al.*, 1992). Sewage sludges are spread on fields or pastures. These sludges contain considerable amounts of heavy metals, persistent organic pollutants, etc. Products from animals grazed on treated areas, or fed on forage or cereals grown on these fields, might contain higher levels of these compounds, depending on crop and animal management systems.
- High levels of dioxins, in milk from cows grazing near incinerators, led to the closure of some of these plants such as three municipal waste incinerators in Lille, France (ENDS daily, 1998), and a chemical waste incinerator belonging to Coalite Chemicals near Bolsover in 1991 (ENDS report, 1997; MAFF, 1997a), or tighter regulations (e.g. British Steel Engineering Steels in the Rotherham area (MAFF, 1997b).
- Recently, contaminated citrus pulp from Brazil, fed to cows in Germany, led to high levels of dioxins in the milk (Malisch, 1998; Malisch *et al.*, 1999; Brooks *et al.*, 1999; Carvalhaes *et al.*, 1999). The citrus pulp was found in the Netherlands, Belgium and the UK as well. The source of the contamination was traced back to lime from a chemical plant that was used to manufacture the lime milk which was subsequently applied in the production of the citrus pulp pellets.

## 5. Conclusions

This topic is very complex, due to the high number of compounds, the multitude of waste types that contribute to emissions into the environment and the high variety of pathways leading to contamination of the food chain and health effects in wildlife, domestic animals and humans. To focus interest on only a selection of hazards means simplifying the problem and reduces the list of substances that industry and governments have to deal with, such as currently polychlorinated dibenzodioxins and incineration, while in the meantime, other compounds are released unmonitored and might cause similar or worse problems. Scientists, farmers, chemists, engineers, doctors and the public should be aware of the complexity of the field and a multidisciplinary approach should be made to avoid feed and consequently food contamination.

Persistent bio-accumulative substances remain stable in the environment and in living organisms. Degradation and metabolism occur very slowly. This means that once an amount of a persistent substance has been produced, it will be released into the environment, unless there is some means of recovery and/or destruction which does not lead to other toxic compounds being formed, such as dioxins and furans. Persistent compounds can be released, either while being produced or used in their application, or later when they are disposed of as waste. The security of the disposal method will mainly have an effect on the speed of release (via leakage, low temperature burning, diffusion, dissolving, volatilisation) and less so on the quantity released.

Increasing the cost of and security of waste treatment will tend to lead to illegal waste disposal (nationally or internationally) and is therefore likely to increase the speed of releases into the environment. As little as a gram of many of these substances can lead to contamination of millions of cubic meters of water, air or soil. Actually, the Belgian scandal was caused by one gram of dioxins and caused more than 2 billion ECUs of economic damage solely in Belgium (Bernard *et al.*, 1999; Hens, 1999).

Regulation of waste treatment, i.e. an end of pipe approach, means dealing with the end of life route for a product, including the route of final disposal. Applying the precautionary principle, which has been agreed to within EU countries, would mean beginning at the other end of the life-cycle, i.e. stopping production. In some applications this might be easily achieved, because they are not deemed to be essential. In other applications, there might be substances or techniques available as alternatives. If not, research on alternatives has to be encouraged and, in the meantime, the production and release has to be minimised, by

- firstly, determining concentrations/amounts that are unavoidable;
- secondly, complex mixtures like most of these polyhalogenated compounds should be replaced by single compound products;
- thirdly, choosing methods, which minimise leakage during usage.

Phasing out and destruction of hazardous substances should be conducted on a short and realistically strict time schedule, not permitting multiple exceptions to the rule, as has occurred in the past (e.g. PCBs).

An adequate safety testing system should be developed prior to marketing. This should include waste treatment during production, use and end of life. Testing should be applied to substances already in use and to newly-developed ones. When substances have to be replaced, arguments for and against should be considered for every application and compound, including the full product life cycle from production process to waste treatment. Whole-life environmental cost-benefit evaluation models must be developed, to enable effective decision-making.

Setting maximum concentrations and allowing 'dilute and disperse' strategies are adequate for substances of acute toxicity with an established NOAEL (no observed adverse effect level) that are rapidly degraded in the environment.

However, the release of persistent bio-accumulative substances with high lipophilicity and low-dose chronic toxicity should be additionally regulated, by setting maximum levels of absolute input into the environment and the aim should be reduction to zero. The policy of 'dilute and disperse' is unacceptable at any level (contaminated product; emission from industry/waste sites into water, air, soil; animal feed, foods).

There is insufficient data on brominated compounds, as well as the formation of brominated and mixed dioxins, furans and biphenyls in fires, incinerator emissions, etc. and further substances that were widely introduced to replace PCBs, e.g. chlorinated alkanes. Monitoring of these compounds, which are not yet regulated, should be implemented. This should assess levels in the environment, food and humans, to establish the relevant trends.

There are still multiple sources of contamination of animal feed and human food, under current waste management strategies. Therefore an effective food control system is still needed to protect the consumer. This should also include those persistent organic pollutants of which levels are known to be currently declining in the environment. Feed quality should comply with the same control measures as food. When contaminated feed stuffs are found, the contaminant should be removed (from the feed or with the feed) and destroyed, to avoid it being sold elsewhere. In Germany, regulation for residues of pesticides has been changed accordingly.

Processes that might increase the contamination of feed, and therefore human food, should be avoided. The aim should be 'levels as low as possible' and not 'contamination up to but not exceeding the TDI (Tolerable Daily Intake)', because actual levels in humans and animals that have occurred under the latter management system are already responsible for measurable effects.

In the light of the recent food scandals involving Brazilian citrus pulp pellets and the Belgian recycled oil for animal feed, we should reconsider the current practice of using animal feed as a route of waste disposal. In the first case lime milk was produced from lime originating from processes in chemical industry; in the second case oil from industrial cooking was being collected and used for animal feed. As far as they went, both practices were carried out on a legal and widely-accepted level. Using waste in food production carries a higher risk of contamination, either accidentally or illegally. Illegal disposal of PCB-transformer oil into the industrial cooking oil led to the feed contamination in the Belgian case.

Considering the special problem that bio-accumulative persistent organic pollutants pose: is the risk caused by using 'waste' (as defined in this chapter) in animal feed still acceptable? Should the precautionary principle be implemented instead, meaning that 'waste' has to be excluded from the food chain or at least undergo strict and dense controls as part of the production and quality control process with producer liability. That would surely result in far more expensive food production. Or can we deal with this problem by adapting the old system of tolerance levels and random controls to the new situation?

Finally we want to repeat that the aim for every regulation for the input of these substances to the environment should be levels **as low as is achievable**. International co-operation on a global scale will be necessary, if we are to reduce and stop the production, release and cycling of these persistent compounds.

At the time of going to press, as if to emphasise the main points in this chapter, reports have been circulating of the routine (and probably illegal) addition of sewage sludge to animal feed in Belgium, France, Germany and the Netherlands (Sunday Telegraph, No 2002, 24th October 1999). In view of the comments above on the contamination of sewage sludge with heavy metals, persistent organic pollutants and other contaminants including viruses, this emphasises the urgent need to regulate and monitor animal feedstuff production on a European-wide basis. The more we look into the animal feed industry the more it is found that it is being used, either knowingly or unwittingly, as a sink for the disposal of unwanted wastes. Readers should appreciate that the main target group for health damage from such practices is the human race.

## References

Aguilar, A., and Borrell, A. (1994) Abnormally high polychlorinated biphenyl levels in striped dolphins (Stenella coeruleoalba) affected by the 1990-1992 Mediterranean epizootic, *Sci. Tot. Environ.* **154**, 237-247.

Allen, Y., Matthiessen, P., Scott, A.P., Haworth, S., Feist, S., and Thain, J.E. (1999) The extent of oestrogenic contamination in the UK estuarine and marine environments - further surveys of flounder, *Sci. Tot. Environ.* **233 (1-3)**, 5-20.

AMAP (1998) AMAP Assessment Report: Arctic pollution issues, Arctic Monitoring and Assessment Programme (AMAP), Oslo, Norway, 859 pp.

Ayotte, P., Dewailly, E., Bruneau, S., Careau, H., and Vezina, A. (1995) Arctic air pollution and human health: what effects should be expected? *Sci. Tot. Environ.* **160-161**, 529-537.

Ayotte, P., Carrier, G., and Dewailly, E. (1996) Health risk assessment for Inuit newborn exposed to dioxin-like compounds through breast-feeding, *Chemosphere* **32** **(3)**, 531-542.

Beck, H., Dross, A., and Mathar, W. (1992) PCDDs, PCDFs, and related contaminants in the German food-supply, *Chemosphere* **25** **(7-10)**, 1539-1550.

Bergman, A., and Olsson, M. (1985) Pathology of Baltic grey seal and ringed seal females with special reference to adrenocortical hyperplasia: is environmental pollution the cause of a widely distributed disease syndrome? *Finnish Game Research* **44**, 47-62.

Bernard, A., Hermans, C., Broeckaert, F., De Poorter, G., De Cock, A., and Houins, G. (1999) Food contamination by PCBs and dioxins, *Nature* **401**, 231-232.

Birmingham, B., Gilman, A., Grant, D., Salminen, J., Boddington, M., Thorpe, B., Wile, I., Toft, P., and Armstrong, V. (1989a) PCDD PCDF multi-media exposure analysis of the Canadian population – Detailed exposure estimation, *Chemosphere* **19** **(1-6)**, 637-642.

Birmingham, B., Thorpe, B., Frank, R., Clement, R., Tosine, H., Fleming, G., Ashman, J., Wheeler, J., Ripley, B.D., and Ryan, J.J. (1989b) Dietary-intake of PCDD and PCDF from food in Ontario, Canada, *Chemosphere* **19** **(1-6)**, 507-512.

Blais, J.M., Schindler, D.W., Muir, D.C.G., Kimpe, L.E., Donald, D.B., and Rosenberg, B. (1998) Accumulation of persistent organochlorine compounds in mountains of western Canada, *Nature* **395** **(6702)**, 585-588.

Bletchly, J.D. (1984) Polychlorinated biphenyls: Production, current use and possible range of future disposal in OECD member countries, in M.C. Barros, H. Konemann and R. Visser (eds), *Proceedings of PCB-Seminar*, Ministry of Housing, Physical Planning and Environment, the Netherlands, pp. 272-343.

Brevik, E.M., Biseth, A., and Oehme, M. (1990) Levels of polychlorinated dibenzofurans and dibenzo-p-dioxins in crude and processed fish oils in relation to origin and cleaning method, 10th Symposium on Halogenated Environmental Organic Pollutants, *Dioxin'90* **1**, 467-470.

Brooks, P., Carvalhaes, G., and Krauss, T. (1999) Chlorinated components in lime used in production of contaminated citrus pulp pellets from Brazil, 19$^{th}$ International Symposium on Halogenated Environmental Organic Pollutants and POPs, *Dioxin'99* **41**, 19-23.

Carvalhaes, G., Brooks, P., and Krauss, T. (1999) Lime as the source of PCDD/F contamination in citrus pulp pellets from Brazil, 19th International Symposium on Halogenated Environmental Organic Pollutants and POPs, *Dioxin'99* **41**, 137-140.

Cuijpers, C.E.J., Bremmer, H.J., Luijckx, N.B.L., van Zorge, J.A., and Liem, A.K.D. (1998) Dioxins and PCBs in the Netherlands. 18th Symposium on Halogenated Environmental Organic Pollutants, *Dioxin'98* **38**, 59-64.

DeGuise, S., Martineau, D., Beland, P., and Fournier, M. (1995) Possible mechanism of action of environmental contaminants on St-Lawrence Beluga whales (Delphinapterus leucas). *Environ. Health Perspect.* **103 (S4)**, 73-77.

Dewailly, E., Ryan, J.J., Laliberte, C., Bruneau, S., Weber, J.P., and Gingras, S. (1994) Exposure of remote maritime populations to coplanar PCBs, *Environ. Health Perspect* **102 (suppl. 1)**, 205-209.

DFG - Deutsche Forschungsgemeinschaft (1997) Potentielle Schadorganismen und Stoffe in Futtermitteln sowie in tierischen Fäkalien, Präsentation des Sachstandsberichtes der Arbeitsgruppe 'Beurteilung von potentiellen Schadorganismen und Stoffen in Futtermitteln sowie tierischen Fäkalien' der DFG-Senatskommission zur Beurteilung von Stoffen in der Landwirtschaft. DFG, Bonn, Germany. (in German)

Duignan, P.J., House, C., Odell, D.K., Wells, R.S., Hansen, L.J., Walsh, M.T., StAubin, D.K., Rima, B.K., and Geraci, J.R. (1996) Morbillivirus infection in bottlenose dolphins: Evidence for recurrent epizootics in the western Atlantic and Gulf of Mexico, *Marine Mammal Science* **12 (4)**, 499-515.

ENDS daily (1998) Dioxin alert shuts French incinerators, *ENDS daily* 29/1/98.

ENDS report (1993) Sludge to land study raises fears about PCBs in food chain, *ENDS report* **242**, Environmental Data Services Ltd. (Publishers).

ENDS report (1997) Dioxins in milk increase near Coalite woks, *ENDS report* **271**, Environmental Data Services Ltd. (Publishers).

ENS (1998) Pharmaceuticals create drinking water headache, *Environment News Service* 23/3/1998.

Fries, G.F. (1996) Ingestion of sludge applied organic chemicals by animals, *Sci. Total Environ.* **185 (1-3)**, 93-108.

Gilbertson, M. (1989) Effects on fish and wildlife populations. in Kimbrough, R.D., and Jensen, A.A. (eds) (1989) *Halogenated Biphenyls, Terphenyls, Naphthalenes, Dibenzodioxins and Related Products*, 2nd ed., Elsevier Science Publishers B.V. (Biomedical Division), Amsterdam, New York, Oxford.

Gilbertson, M., Kubiak, T., Ludwig, J., and Fox, G. (1991) Great Lakes embryo mortality, edema, and deformities syndrome (GLEMEDS) in colonial fish-eating birds: similarity to chick-edema disease, *J. Toxicol. Environ. Health* **33**, 455-520.

Grachev, M.A., Kumarev, V.P., Mamaev, L.V., Zorin, V.L., Baranova, L.V., Denikina, N.N., Belikov, S.I., Petrov, E.A., Kolesnik, V.S., Kolesnik, R.S., Dorofeev, V.M., Beim, A.M., Kudelin, V.N., Nagieva, F.G., and Sidorov, V.N. (1989) Distemper virus in Baikal seals, *Nature* **238**, 209.

Grandjean, P., Weihe, P., Needham, L.L., Burse, V.W., Patterson, D.G., and Sampson, E.J. (1995) Relation of a seafood diet to mercury, selenium, arsenic, and polychlorinated biphenyl and other organochlorine concentrations in human milk, *Environ. Res.* **71** (**1**), 29-38.

Greenpeace (1999) Newsletter for Germany 4/98-1/99.

Gülden, M., Turan, A., and Seibert, H. (1997) Substanzen mit endokriner Wirkung in Oberflächengewässern, Umweltbundesamt [Substances with Endocrine Activity in Surface Waters, Environmental Protection Agency], Forschungsbericht 102 04 279, UBA-FB 97-068, Texte 46/97. UBA, Berlin, Germany. (in German)

Harries, J.E., Sheahan, D.A., Jobling, S., Matthiessen, P., Neall, M., Sumpter, J.P., Taylor, T., and Zaman, N. (1997) Estrogenic activity in five United Kingdom rivers detected by measurement of vitellogenesis in caged male trout, *Environmental Toxicology and Chemistry* **16** (**3**), 534-542.

Harries, J.E., Janbakhsh, A., Jobling, S., Matthiessen, P., Sumpter, J.P., and Tyler, C.R. (1999) Estrogenic potency of effluent from two sewage treatment works in the United Kingdom, *Environmental Toxicology and Chemistry* **18** (**5**), 932-937.

Harwood, J. (1998) What killed monk seals? *Nature* **393**, 17-18.

HAZ (1998) local newspaper Hannoverische Allgemeine Zeitung Oct. 1998.

Heide-Jørgensen, M.P., and Reeves, R.R. (1996) Evidence of a decline in beluga, Delphinapterus leucas, abundance off West Greenland, *ICES J. Marine Science* **53** (**1**), 61-72.

Heide-Jørgensen, M.P., Härkönen, T., Dietz, R., and Thompson, P.M. (1992) Retrospective of the 1988 European seal epizootic, *Dis. Aquat. Org.* **13**, 37-62.

Helle, E. (1981) Reproductive trends and occurrence of organochlorines and heavy metals in the Baltic seal populations, *ICES. C.M.* 1981/E:37.

Hens, L. (1999) Dioxines en PCBs in Belgische eieren en kippen, *Milieu* **14** (**4**), 220-224. (in Dutch)

Hernandez, M., Robinson, I., Aguilar, A., Gonzalez, L.M., Lopez-Jurado, L.F., Reyero, M.I., Cacho, E., Franco, J., Lopez-Rodas, V., Costas, E. (1998) Did algal toxins cause monk seal mortality? *Nature* **393**, 28-29.

International Environment Reporter (1998) Polychlorinated biphenyls: United States announces agreement to accelerate PCB phaseout in Russia, vol. 21, no. 14, p. 668.

Isosaari, P., Hallikainen, A., Ruohonen, K., and Vartiainen, T. (1998) Concentrations of PCDD/Fs and PCBs in rainbow trout fed with Baltic herring and dry fish feed, 18th Symposium on Halogenated Environmental Pollutants, *Dioxin'98*, Stockholm, Sweden, **39**, 393-396.

Jacobs, M.N., and Johnston, P.A. (1995) Organochlorine pesticide and PCB residues in pharmaceutical and industrial grade fish oils, Greenpeace Research Laboratories, University of Exeter, Technical Note 05/96, 4, May 1995.

Kannan, K., Tanabe, S., Borrell, A., Aguilar, A., Focardi, S., and Tatsukawa, R. (1993) Isomer-specific analysis and toxic evaluation of polychlorinated biphenyls in striped dolphins affected by an epizootic in the Western Mediterranean Sea, *Arch. Environ. Contam. Toxicol.* **25**, 227-233.

Kidd, K.A., Schindler, D.W., Muir, D.C.G., Lockhart, W.L., and Hesslein, R.H. (1995) High concentrations of toxaphene in fishes from a subarctic lake, *Science* **269 (5221)**, 240-242.

Kimbrough, R.D., and Jensen, A.A. (eds) (1989) *Halogenated Biphenyls, Terphenyls, Naphthalenes, Dibenzodioxins and Related Products*, 2nd ed., Elsevier Science Publishers B.V. (Biomedical Division), Amsterdam, New York, Oxford.

Lair, S., Beland, P., DeGuise, S., and Martineau, D. (1997) Adrenal hyperplastic and degenerative changes in Beluga whales, *Journal of Wildlife Diseases* **33 (3)**, 430-437.

Liem, A.K.D. (1999) Dioxins and dioxin-like PCBs in foodstuffs. Levels and trends, *Organohalogen Compounds* **44**, 1-4.

Liem, A.K.D., and Theelen, R.M.C. (1997) Dioxins: chemical analysis, exposure and risk assessment, Thesis, Utrecht University, ISBN 90-393-2012-8.

Lund, B.O. (1994) In vitro adrenal bioactivation and effects on steroid metabolism of DDT, PCBs and their metabolites in the Gray seal (Halichoerus grypus), *Environmental Toxicology and Chemistry* **13 (6)**, 911-917.

MAFF (1997a) Food Surveillance Sheet 124: Dioxins and PCBs in cows' milk from the Bolsover area.

MAFF (1997b) Food Surveillance Sheet 123: Dioxins and PCBs in cows' milk from farms close to industrial sites: 1996 survey results.

MAFF (1997c) Food Surveillance Sheet 106 Dioxins and Polychlorinated Biphenyls in Fish Oil Dietary Supplements and Licensed Medicines.

Malisch, R. (1998) Increase of PCDD/F-contamination of milk and butter in Germany by use of contaminated citrus pulps as component in feed, 18th Symposium on Halogenated Environmental Organic Pollutants, *Dioxin'98* **38**, 65-70.

Malisch, R., Berger, B., and Verstraete, F. (1999) Lime as source for PCDD/F-contamination of Brazilian citrus pulp pellets (CPPs), 19th International Symposium on Halogenated Environmental Organic Pollutants and POPs, *Dioxin'99* **41**, 51-53.

Marquenie, J.M., and Reijnders, P.J.H. (1989) PCBs, an increasing concern for the marine environment, *ICES. C.M.* 1989/N:12.

Mason, C.F. (1998) Decline in PCB levels in Otters (Lutra lutra), *Chemosphere* **36 (9)**, 1969-1971.

McLachlin, M.S., Hinkel, M., Reissinger, M., Kaupp, H., Hippelein, M., and Hutzinger, O. (1992) Klärschlammdüngung - Eintrag von PCDD, PCDF und PCB in die Nahrungskette, Bayerisches Staatsministerium für Landesentwicklung und Umweltfragen (eds, publisher), München, Germany. (in German)

Mengelers, M.J.B., Hoogenboom, L.A.P., and Traag, W.A. (1999) State of affairs with regard to the dioxin contamination of animal feed in Belgium (the Belgian dioxin affair), 19th International Symposium on Halogenated Environmental Organic Pollutants and POPs, *Dioxin'99,* only on cd-rom version of the Proceedings.

Montague, P. (1998) Frogs, alligators and pesticides, *Rachel's Environment and Health Weekly* **590** (whole issue, http://www.rachel.org/).

Oetjen, K., and Karl, H. (1997) Herkunft der Toxaphenbelastung von gefarmten Fischen, *Lebensmittelchemie* **51**, 95. (in German)

Ozalla, M.D., To-Figueras, J., Herrero, C., Sala, M., Sunyer, J., Otero, R., and Grimalt, J. (1998) Porphyrin analysis in a human population highly exposed to hexachlorobenzene, 18th symposium on Halogenated Environmental Organic Pollutants, *Dioxin'98* **38**, 151-154.

Patandin, S. (1999) Effects of environmental exposure to polychlorinated biphenyls and dioxins on growth and development in young children, PhD Thesis, Erasmus University, Rotterdam, Microweb, Saasveld, the Netherlands, ISBN 90-9012306-7.

Purdom, C.E., Hardiman, P.A., Bye, V.J., Eno, N.C., Tyler, C.R., and Sumpter, J.P. (1994) Oestrogenic effects of effluent from sewage treatment works, *Chemistry & Ecology* **8**, 275-285.

Reijnders, P.J.H., and Brasseur, S.M.J.M. (1992) Xenobiotic induced hormonal and associated developmental disorders in marine organisms and related effects in humans: an overview, in T. Colborn, and C. Clement (eds), Chemically induced alterations in sexual and functional development: The wildlife/human connection, *Advances in Modern Environmental Toxicology* **11**, Princetown Scientific Publishers Co. Inc., Princetown, USA, pp. 159-174.

Simmonds, M.P., Johnston, P.A., and French, M.C. (1993) Organochlorine and mercury contamination in United Kingdom seals, *The Veterinary Record* **132**, 291-295.

Stringer, R.L., Jacobs, M.N., Johnston, P.A., Wyatt, C.L., Santillo, D. (1996) Organochlorine residues in fish oil dietary supplements, 16th Symposium on Halogenated Environmental Organic Pollutants, *Dioxin'96* **28**, 551-556.

Sumpter, J.P., and Jobling, S. (1995) Vitellogenesis as a biomarker for oestrogenic contamination of the aquatic environment, *Environ. Health Perspect.* **103**, 172-178.

Swedish EPA (1998) *Persistent Organic Pollutants - A Swedish View of an International Problem*, (monitor 16), Swedish Environmental Protection Agency, Stockholm, Sweden.

Tanabe, S. (1988) PCB problems in the future: Foresight from current knowledge, *Environmental Pollution* **50**, 5-28.

Tanabe, S., Iwata, H., and Tatsukawa, R. (1994) Global contamination by persistent organochlorines and their ecotoxicological impact on marine mammals, *The Science of the Total Environment* **154**, 163-177.

Theelen, R.M.C. (1991) Biological basis for risk assessment of dioxins and related compounds, in M.A. Gallo, R.J. Scheuplein, and K.A. van der Heijden (eds), *Banbury Report 35*, Cold Spring Harbor Laboratory Press, p. 277.

Umweltbundesamt - UBA (1989) Sachstand Polybromierte Dibenzodioxine, Polybromierte Dibenzofurane [Environmental Protection Agency (1989) Report on Polybrominated Dibenzodioxins, Polybrominated Dibenzofurans], UBA, Berlin, Germany. (in German)

van Birgelen, A.P.J.M. (1998) Hexachlorobenzene as a possible major contributor to the dioxin activity of human milk, *Environ. Health Perspectives* **106 (11)**, 683-688.

Wiig, O., Derocher, A.E., Cronin, N.M., and Skaare, J.U. (1998) Female pseudohermaphrodite polar bears at Svalbard, *Journal of Wildlife Diseases* **34** (**4**), 792-796.

# TOWARDS A PRECAUTIONARY APPROACH FOR WASTE MANAGEMENT SUPPORTED BY EDUCATION AND INFORMATION TECHNOLOGY


L. HENS[1]
P. NICOLOPOULOU-STAMATI[2]
C.V. HOWARD[3]
J. LAFERE[1]
G. STAATS DE YANES[4]

*[1]Vrije Universiteit Brussel*
*Human Ecology Department*
*Laarbeeklaan 103*
*B-1090 Brussel*
*BELGIUM*

*[2]National and Capodistrian University of Athens*
*Medical School, Department of Pathology*
*75, Micres Ajias, GOYDI*
*11527 Athens*
*GREECE*

*[3]University of Liverpool*
*Fetal & Infant Toxico-Pathology*
*P.O. Box 147*
*L69 7ZA Liverpool*
*UNITED KINGDOM*

*[4]WHO-Centre*
*Tierärztlichen Hochschule Hannover*
*Bünteweg 2*
*D-30559 Hannover*
*GERMANY*




*P. Nicolopoulou-Stamati et al. (eds.), Health Impacts of Waste Management Policies,* 283–310.

## Summary

This chapter concludes the information provided in these proceedings. The state of the art of the knowledge on health hazards associated with waste deposit sites and incinerators is overviewed. In particular cancers, congenital malformations, genetic damage, neurological and behavioural changes, immunological impairment, reproductive failure and interference with hormones seem to be the main health end points of the pollutants involved. These data also point to the fragmentary and *ad hoc* character of this information. Both elements are crucial in the scientific uncertainty which is manifest.

Waste policy in the EU widely accepts the prevention - re-use – recycling - thermal valorisation-controlled disposal hierarchy. Nevertheless, waste disposal and incineration are the prevailing management options in practice. To protect health a significant move towards more prevention and re-use seems most necessary. The conceptual basis for this is embedded in a revived application of the precautionary principle. Health impact assessment, environmental taxes and environmental education might prove to become major instrumental pillars of such a proactive waste policy. An environmental education strategy might be based on the 'Declaration of Kos' advocating training and education for a wide array of target groups including biomedical and environmental experts, an interdisciplinary approach and the installation of a chemical hygiene attitude.


## 1. Introduction

This book discusses the interface between health effects which can result from (inappropriate) waste disposal practices and incineration, and waste policy options.

The health aspects are introduced by a general overview, on the relationship between persistent organic chemicals and the health effects they might cause. This information is complemented by a substance related approach in which particulates are also identified as pollutants. It is important in understanding the health consequences of waste management options. The health picture is completed by the analysis of case studies of open incineration in Amsterdam (the Netherlands) and household waste incineration near Antwerp (Belgium).

The policy aspects are discussed from a twofold viewpoint. The possibilities and limitations of policy instruments such as health risk assessment and their use in environmental impact assessment are addressed next to the prevention capacity of environmental taxes on selected waste streams.

The book also provides a round-up of waste management policies in the European Union, the USA, and in selected EU-member states. Moreover, the attitude of the World Health Organisation and the comments of the European Environmental Technology Industry and those of the European environmental organisations are documented.

This chapter aims at drawing conclusions from this wealth of information along four lines. The **health data** are summarised in a way which overviews the state of the art knowledge on the hazards associated with exposure to pollutants originating from waste deposit sites and incinerators. This overview also shows the extent to which our knowledge is fragmentary and lacks systematics. It also reveals aspects of scientific uncertainty.

The **policy lines** in the different member states of the EU show more and more coherence to the basic principles. The prevention - re-use – recycling - thermal decomposition with energy recovery-controlled disposal hierarchy is accepted universally. This is in line with the main concerns of the World Health Organisation. Interpretations differ, however, e.g. about the contributing capacity of incineration in a sustainable waste policy and the level of the emission standards. This results in an interesting variability in the waste policy options in the different EU member states.

In spite of the consensus about what should be done, the majority of waste in Europe is either land filled or incinerated. These are the methods also entailing the highest health risk. A significant policy move towards waste prevention and re-use can be realised under two conditions:

a. a sound foundation of waste policy on the precautionary principle;
b. more intensive use of policy instruments such as environmental taxes, health impact assessments and environmental education which, if used judiciously, all have a contribution to make towards prevention of harm.

## 2. Health Effects of Waste Management

Pollution resulting from waste deposit sites can reach man and the food chain through leachate which contaminates the surface and the groundwater and through atmospheric emissions. Rare exposure is also mediated directly by exposure through contaminated soil resulting from pica behaviour. Table 39 shows that exposure to air and water pollution by waste deposit sites has been associated with congenital malformations, airway inflammation, gastro-intestinal symptoms, cancer, chromosomal changes, low birthweight, effects on mood, narcotic and skin, and tiredness. However, quantitative data allowing forecasts of health effects for new projects are rare to inexistent. The heterogeneity of both the pollutants and the exposure routes is an important factor underlying this problem.

These studies are retrospective in character. They reflect the medium- and long-term effects of waste deposited decades ago, in accordance with the technologies which were in use at that time. They were considered to be safe and up-to-date at that time, but practice and the appreciation of the associated hazards has changed significantly since then.

*Table 39.* Health effects in populations living near waste deposition sites.[7]

| Site description (project type, location, year of inauguration) | Effects investigated | Results | Reference |
|---|---|---|---|
| 1. Multicentre case-control study (cases = 1089; controls = 2366), which included 21 landfill sites in Europe: 9 closed before the start of study period; 10 were in operation for more than 20 years | Congenital malformations | Increased risk of congenital malformations in babies whose mothers live close to landfill sites | Dolk *et al.*, 1998 |

[7] The data of tables 1 to 4 were selected by using WinSpirs 2.1 (Medline) from 1968 till 1999. The following keywords were inserted and matched: 'health', 'household/deposit site', 'waste', 'landfill site', 'incineration/incinerating', 'recycling' and 'composting'.

*Table 39.* Continued.

| Site description (project type, location, year of inauguration) | Effects investigated | Results | Reference |
|---|---|---|---|
| 2. Case-control analyses near a municipal solid waste landfill site in Montreal (Canada) | Low birthweight and preterm births | Low birthweight incidence was significantly higher in the exposure zone proximal to the site exposed changes. Excess risks were also observed for small for gestational age, but the association was not as strong as for low birthweight | Goldberg *et al*., 1995b |
| 3. Cross sectional and longitudinal studies at a combined industrial/ household waste deposit site in Mellery, Belgium, 1992 | Chromosomal changes (Sister-chromatid exchange, high frequency cell analysis, single-strand breaks, and micro-nucleus test) | Increased incidence of SCE, SSB, MN and HFC, especially in children | Klemans *et al*., 1995<br>Lakhanisky *et al*., 1993<br>Laurent *et al*., 1993 |
| 4. Case-control study on household waste collectors (25 waste collectors; 24 controls)in Kristianstad in southern Sweden | Airway inflammation and general symptoms | Increased risk of airway inflammation, general symptoms (diarrhoea, congested nose, tiredness) in association with higher β-D-glucan levels | Thorn *et al* .,1998 |
| 5. Case control study in waste collectors (1747 male waste collectors, 1111 male municipality workers) in Denmark: season, equipment and job function related to gastro-intestinal problems | Gastro-intestinal problems | Gastro-intestinal symptoms were associated with the job of waste collector and occurred more in summer | Ivens *et al*., 1997 |

*Table 39.* Continued.

| Site description (project type, location, year of inauguration) | Effects investigated | Results | Reference |
|---|---|---|---|
| 6. Case-control study (cases = 197 subjects; controls = 235 subjects) at the Upper Ottawa street landfill site in Hamilton, Ontario, which opened in the early 1950s and closed in 1980 | Mood, narcotic, skin, and respiratory conditions | The vapours, fumes, or particulate matter emanating from the landfill site, as well as direct skin exposure, may have lead to the health effects on mood, narcotic, skin and respiratory conditions found in excess | Hertzman *et al.*, 1987 |
| 7. Case-control studies at a municipal solid waste landfill site in Montreal (Canada) which opened in 1968 | Cancer | Excess risk of cancers of the stomach, trachea, bronchus, lung, liver, kidney, pancreas and non-Hodgkin's lymphomas in men living near the landfill site. Among women, rates of stomach cancer and cervix uteri cancer were increased | Goldberg *et al.*, 1999<br>Goldberg *et al.*, 1995a |
| 8. Incidence study (1978-1985) of a bladder cancer cluster in north-western Illinois (USA), near a landfill site (operating since 1972) | Bladder cancer | Elevated risks of bladder cancer in areas near a landfill site | Mallin, 1990 |

Waste incineration offers a more complex environmental pollution phenomenon. Figure 32 shows the distribution of pollutants emitted by a household waste incineration plant over water, air and soil. Quantitative data on this process are provided in Figure 23. Both this figures show that the released pollutants stem in part from the chemically stable compounds found in the input waste. Different heavy metal compounds provide an example of these. Another portion of the emitted products are synthesised during the incineration process, often after the gases have left the combustion chamber and during the process of cooling them down before they are emitted into the air. Dioxins provide a notorious example of this. Dioxins and related products present in the original waste, largely as a result of anthropogenic activities such as incineration, are (partly) destroyed in the oven. They are, however, abundantly reformed *'de novo'* during the treatment of the oven gasses. Most incinerators limit the dioxin emissions by treating the gasses with activated carbon which, provided the delivery system is working to specification, absorbs an appreciable part of the persistent chemicals, before the emissions are released into the atmosphere.

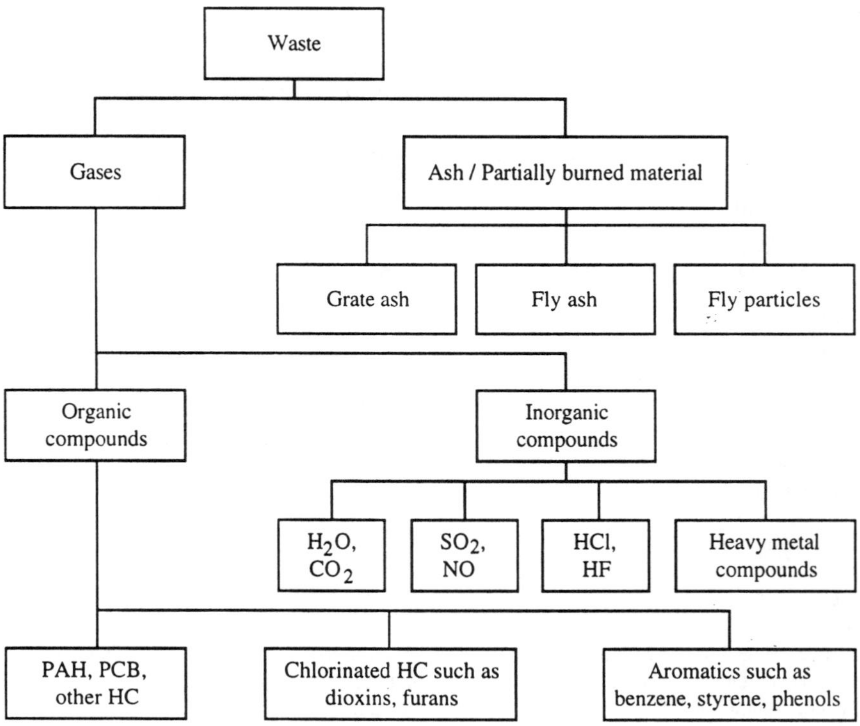


*Figure 32.* The distribution of pollutants emitted by a household waste incineration plant over the environmental compartments.

Waste incineration is also complex because the pollutants are dispersed as a solid (grate and fly ashes), a water (spargate) and an air fraction. The solid fraction is either land filled or further treated. The water fraction is, eventually after treatment, released into the environment. The same applies for the emissions into the atmosphere. The overall result is effectively a dilution and dispersion of pollution both in space and over time. This causes a slow but gradual accumulation in the food chain and the human body, so that effects become visible and measurable only after a long latency period.

Even in this complex environmental context of emission, transport, transformation and exposure, populations living near incinerators have been reported to show increased incidences of chromosomal changes, congenital malformations, cancer, respiratory diseases, and effects on the immune system (Table 40). Scarce relative risk figures indicate that cancer risks might be elevated by a factor 6,7.

*Table 40.* Health effects in populations living near incineration plants.

| Site description (project type, location, year of inauguration) | Effects investigated | Results | Reference |
|---|---|---|---|
| 1. Open incineration industrial waste Rotterdam, The Netherlands, 1968 | Congenital malformations | Increased risk of orofacial clefts | Ten Tusscher *et al.*, 2000 |
| 2. Geographical birth registration in an area (= Falkirk district) with 2 incineration plants in central Scotland. Both incinerators had ceased operating before the study began | Sex ratios of births | Statistically significant excesses of female births | Williams *et al.*, 1992 |
| 3. Retrospective health study and cytogenic study of a population living near a household waste incineration Wilrijk, Belgium, 1998 | Chromosomal aberrations<br>Congenital malformations<br>Multiple pregnancies<br>Learning problems | Increased rate of multiple pregnancies – no statistical significant increase of other parameters | Van Larebeke, 2000 |
| 4. A 10-year follow-up in inhabitants (n = 179) living in the vicinity of a hazardous waste incinerator (1984-1994) in Riihimäki, Finland | Mercury poisoning | Mercury exposure increased as distance from the plant decreased, however, the increase in exposure was minimal and did not pose a health risk | Kurttio *et al.*, 1998 |

*Table 40.* Continued.

| Site description (project type, location, year of inauguration) | Effects investigated | Results | Reference |
|---|---|---|---|
| 5. Dioxin analysis in non-occupationally exposed persons living in the vicinity of a municipal waste incinerator in Schwandorf (Germany) | Dioxin levels in blood and human milk | No indication of enhanced body burden of PCDD/F; no direct health hazards | Deml *et al.*, 1996 |
| 6. Internal exposure of industrial waste incineration workers in Germany | Higher internal exposure to organic and inorganic substances | The biological exposure limits valid in Germany were not exceeded in any cases | Wrbitzky *et al.*, 1995 |
| 7. Mortality risk analysis in area of Malagrotta (Rome, Italy) with large waste disposal site, incinerator and oil refinery plant | Standardised mortality ratios for several cancers (liver, lung, lympho-haematopoietic, and laryngeal) | No association between proximity to industrial sites and mortality. Laryngeal cancer declined with distance from the sources of pollution | Michelozzi *et al.*, 2000 |
| 8. Incidence study of 72 municipal solid waste incinerators in Great Britain | Cancer | A statistically significant decline in risk with distance from incinerators for all cancers combined stomach, colorectal, liver and lung cancer | Elliott *et al.*, 1996 |
| 9. Cohort study from municipal refuse incinerator workers and water treatment workers, 1990 (3 months) in USA (anonymous) | Mutagens and promutagens (Ames assay) | Increased risk of both mutagens and promutagens in first urine samples of incinerator workers. No difference in $2^{nd}$ and $3^{rd}$ urine samples | Ma *et al.*, 1992 |
| 10. Testing of extracts of airborne particulates collected inside the working area of municipal incinerator of Trieste (Italy) | Mutagenicity test of extracts of airborne dust (Ames assay) | Most samples of dust were proved to be mutagenic. Samples of solid residues collected at the end of the combustion process showed only weak mutagenic response | Pani *et al.*, 1983 |

*Table 40.* Continued.

| Site description (project type, location, year of inauguration) | Effects investigated | Results | Reference |
|---|---|---|---|
| 11. Case-control study (755 case-control pairs) in the area of a household waste incinerator at Trieste (Italy) | Lung cancer | Increased rate of lung cancer incidence (RR = 6,7) | Biggeri *et al.*, 1996 |
| 12. Case-control study of 100 male children 10 years of age on the garbage dumps of Cairo (30% of garbage is burned) | Immune system, allergic respiratory disease | Secretory IgA is strongly affected; higher rate of hyperreactive mucous membranes in exposed children | Marth *et al.*, 1995 |
| 13. Cross sectional study of populations living in the neighbourhood of 3 waste incinerators in North Carolina (US) | Adverse respiratory effects | No increased risk in acute or chronic respiratory symptoms | Shy *et al.*, 1995 |
| 14. Retrospective comparison study in a village of the Isere department (France) near an incinerator (1981). The village was divided in 3 areas (high – low – very low exposure) | Respiratory problems | Increased consumption of medicines for respiratory problems as the distance of the residents' homes from the incinerator decreased | Zmirou *et al.*, 1984 |

This book reports results from the study of new-born babies exposed to dioxins and PCBs transplacentally and through breast milk. Negative effects were found on the development of the thyroid hormone metabolism, psychomotor development, behaviour and the immune system (Koppe *et al.*, 2000).

Open air combustion of industrial waste chemicals in Zeeburg, Amsterdam (the Netherlands) is closely associated with non-syndromal orofacial clefts in new-born babies (ten Tusscher *et al.*, 2000).

Van Larebeke (2000) reports on an increased incidence of multiple pregnancies in a population living near a household waste incinerator in Wilrijk, near Antwerp (Belgium). In the same population the incidence of congenital malformations was increased, although this latter increase was not statistically significant.

Clearly not all the studies summarised in Table 40 show the same effects, but they are all characterised by their specific sensitivity and statistical power.

Nevertheless the global picture which emerges is that cancer, congenital malformations, alterations to genetic material, neurological and neurobehavioural changes, immunologic impairment, reproductive failure and interference with the (thyroid and oestrogen) hormonal balance are the main health effect indices influenced by pollutants from waste deposit sites and incinerators.

In order to reduce the strain on the environment from the deposition of waste in landfills and combustion at incineration plants, several governments throughout the industrialised world have planned greatly increased recycling of domestic waste. The main health problems associated with recycling processes are gastric cancer, musculoskeletal problems, respiratory and pulmonary diseases, ODTS symptoms, gastro-intestinal problems and irritation of eye, skin and mucous membranes. The results are summarised in Table 41.

*Table 41.* Health effects in populations living near recycling facilities.

| **Site description (project type, location, year of inauguration)** | **Effects investigated** | **Results** | **Reference** |
|---|---|---|---|
| 1. Cohort study of male subjects (n = 532) employed at 2 municipal plants for garbage recycling and incinerating in Rome, Italy, which began operating in 1962 | Cancer (lung and gastric) | Mortality from lung cancer was reduced; increased risk was found for gastric cancer (confined in category with more than 10 year since 1st exposure) | Rapiti *et al.*, 1997 |

*Table 41.* Continued.

| Site description (project type, location, year of inauguration) | Effects investigated | Results | Reference |
|---|---|---|---|
| 2. Industrial hygiene measurements (197 measurements) in 6 Danish paper recycling plants (2 closed in 1993) | Exposure to hazardous chemicals | The assessment of chemicals did not reveal a major use of possible carcinogens | Rix *et al* .,1996 |
| 3. Cross-sectional study (596 individuals exposed; 743 individuals unexposed) in the vicinity of a waste recycling plant in Monterrey (Mexico) | Acute and chronic illnesses, problems during pregnancy, congenital illnesses | The most frequently reported health effects were irritation of the eyes and upper respiratory tract, allergies, sleep disturbances, bronchitis, fatigue, skin problems, ear infections, and anaemia. No significant differences in the prevalence of obstetric problems, miscarriages or children born with congenital deformities or low birthweight | Tovalin-Ahumada, 1998 |
| 4. Sorting and recycling of domestic waste: review of occupational health problems | Organic dust toxic syndrome, gastro-intestinal problems, irritation of the skin, eye and mucous membranes of the nose and upper airways | Cross-sectional studies have indicated an excess risk of work-related health problems such as musculoskeletal problems, pulmonary diseases, ODTS symptoms, gastro-intestinal problems and irritation of eye, skin and mucous membranes | Poulsen *et al*., 1995 |
| 5. Field bioassay of a river heavily polluted with paper recycling wastes (eastern USA) | Chromosomal aberrations in fern populations | High incidence of chromosome mutations | Klekowski *et al*., 1979 |

In composting centres the microbiological quality matters. A main problem here is odour, which can (incompletely) be abated. The main health problems associated with composting activities are fungus infections in the respiratory system and allergic reactions caused by fungal exposure (Table 42). The results, however, are not equivocal.

*Table 42.* Health effects in populations living near composting facilities.

| Site description (project type, location, year of inauguration) | Effects investigated | Results | Reference |
|---|---|---|---|
| 1. Airborne molds and their metabolites at workplaces in composting plants | Allergic effects | Not known: lack of information an the toxicological impact of MVOC | Fischer *et al.*, 1998 |
| 2. Case report study of a man living in the neighbourhood of a municipal leaf compost site | Allergic bronchopulmonary aspergillosis | Inhalation of Aspergillus fumigatus spores liberated from a municipal leaf compost site led to the development of ABPA in a patient living in the area | Kramer *et al.*, 1989 |
| 3. Hazard to man and the environment caused by the use of urban waste compost: a review | Lung damage and allergies | Unclear because of scarce data | Deportes *et al* .,1995 |
| 4. Ambient aerospora monitoring and air sampling from municipal sewage sludge composting operations in the state of Maine (US) | Public health risks due to elevated A. fumigatus aerospora concentrations | Residents in the vicinity of the composting operations were not exposed to increased concentrations of A. fumigatus aerospora | Passman, 1983 |

Waste deposit sites, incinerators and recycling facilities release a wide array of pollutants into the environment. Persistent organic chemicals including dioxins, furans and PCBs have received due attention. The health effect of heavy metals in environmental concentrations were also studied in depth. The attention paid by the environmental health researchers to small particulates is more recent. But environmental health research about the bulk of pollutants emitted in these complex cocktails of substances still remains almost non-existent. Equally unknown are the interactive (synergistic, antagonistic, additive) effects which happen during the complex process of transport and transformation through the environment and in the human body.

This lack of information is illustrative of the fragmentary knowledge of health effects and environmental exposure conditions. These fragments in combination with their *ad hoc* character (the reasons why particular situations are studied are merely found in the social-political context of the problem rather than in its scientific importance), provide an important source of scientific uncertainty. Moreover, the *post factum* aspect of most situations results in the understanding of effects generated by situations prevailing one or more decades ago. In the meantime techniques, regulations and attitudes have changed. Therefore these hazard data are limited in their capacity to predict the health effects of new projects, adjusted policies and waste management plans and programmes. Nevertheless they clarify the existing reality of those occurring health problems which are mainly associated with waste deposit sites and incinerators.

## 3. Policy Options on Waste Management

Driven by EU-Directives (Linher, 2000), the main policy lines in the EU member states show increasing coherence. The waste management hierarchy in which prevention prevails over re-use, recycling, thermal treatment (of which incineration is currently the most important) with energy recuperation and controlled disposal, is accepted widely. Differences exist, however, when this hierarchy is implemented in practice:

a. the incineration industry claims that the negative environmental impacts of household waste incineration are exaggerated and that insufficient attention is paid to the environmental benefits of this technology (Lindbauer, 2000);
b. environmental organisations disagree with the Commission on emission standards for incinerators and indeed on the whole concept of incineration of waste as a sustainable activity (Vardaka-Sotiropoulos, 2000);
c. authorities interpret the hierarchy in a flexible way. While Austria and Switzerland incinerate more than 50 per cent of their household waste, Greece has opted for composting. This option is based upon a combination of environmental, feasibility and financial arguments (Dontas, 2000).

The theory of the waste management hierarchy sharply contrasts with the practice. At this moment 60 per cent of household waste throughout the Union is deposited in landfills. In candidate member states such as Poland, this proportion increases to 99 per cent. In addition, in the US the amount of waste deposited has remained fairly constant during the last twenty years. Increasing quantities have been incinerated while selective sorting and recycling has mainly been left to voluntary initiatives (Valaoras, 2000).

It is noteworthy that the waste management hierarchy used in the EU is not rooted in environmental health data. However, it should also be noted that the available data on health effects do not conflict, and in important aspects even coincide, with the hierarchy. A particular aspect of this is the WHO's opposition to uncontrolled waste dumps which are considered as generators of disease, in favour of options ranking higher in the management hierarchy (Rushbrook, 2000).

The question arises, then, as to how to move away from the health-threatening landfill and incineration practices and how to move towards more prevention and re-use. Two aspects of environmental waste policy might prove to have a key role: the precautionary principle and a mix of instruments aimed at making prevention effective.

## 4. A More Precautionary Approach for Waste Management

Policy decisions need to be based on the best available scientific evidence (Brundtland, 1999). Although we have increasing knowledge on the health impacts of waste management, which is of use in policy decisions, nevertheless, scientific uncertainty is problematic. Basically, we are in a situation where different studies point to health problems and act as warning signs. Such a scenario should not result in governmental inactivity, rather decisions should be taken which implement the precautionary principle.

The precautionary principle holds that where there are threats of serious or irreversible danger, lack of full scientific certainty shall not be used as a reason for postponing cost-efficiency measures to prevent environmental degradation. Expressed more liberally, when in doubt about the impact of a development, it will be managed according to the worst-case scenario of its impact on the environment and human health (Hens, 1996).

It should be noted that in the discussion on the health impacts of waste management policies all conditions for the application of the precautionary principle are fulfilled:

- the health effects associated with uncontrolled disposal and incineration are most serious; as far as e.g. damage to DNA is concerned, they are also almost irreversible;
- the subject is a matter of scientific uncertainty and full evidence is lacking;
- cost-effective measures are possible as is shown e.g. by the Greek policy option to treat more than 50 per cent of household waste by composting rather than through incineration.

Applying the precautionary principle in cases of pervasive technologies (these are activities that can affect the quality of life by imprinting upon general public health, as in the case of incinerators or waste deposit sites, but also, e.g. in the case of the release of genetically modified organisms, as discussed e.g. by Howard and Saunders (1999) in their refutation of Holm and Harris, 1999) is not only a matter for the authorities who must act with caution, which is to say on the balance of possibilities rather than with absolute proof; developers must have the onus put upon them to show that their technology is safe rather than society forever having to try to prove that it is unsafe, usually after widespread release of the technology. Evidence of safety must be based upon realistic and relevant hazard assessment and not on fact-free risk assessments. Furthermore, strict liability should apply with pervasive technologies.

It remains a fact that one of the major tools employed by industry and regulators to avoid having to invoke the precautionary principle continues to be the use of unrealistic risk assessments, applied to complex systems, where it is not even possible in many cases to formulate the correct questions with regard to hazard, let alone set about testing them.

We now provide an example of the inappropriate use of risk assessment, by the application of criteria which, though apparently suitable for transient pollutants, can clearly be seen to be inadequate when applied to persistent pollutants.

For substances that remain in the body, even after the environmental level has fallen, the approach of simply setting emission limits is unlikely to succeed in protecting human health. A typical risk assessment for an aerial pollutant from a plant, for example a municipal waste incinerator, will take into account the maximal concentration of a persistent organic pollutant in the plume, such as dioxin. A terrain dispersion model is used to estimate the maximum ground level concentration. Note that at this stage in the risk assessment process, not a single piece of real data will have been used. In environmental risk assessments, there is often an accompanying calculation of the theoretical amount of the pollutant which an adult, standing at the point of maximum ground level concentration for 20 years, might expect to assimilate, while eating food produce grown at that spot. For an example of such an application see Bridges (1992). This approach is always accompanied by an unstated model assumption; namely that the said modelled adult is free from any pollutant in his body at the start of the exercise and that there are no other sources. This is a classical example of inadequate hazard identification. In reality (see Chapter 'Persistent Organic Chemical Pollution: An Introduction') human body burdens of pollutants such as the dioxin-like substances are already acknowledged to be too high.

Therefore the use of empirical dispersion models, presented as an assurance of lack of risk to health, cannot suffice with bio-accumulative persistent toxic substances. Essential additional information is required, over and above what is used in the assessment of transient pollutants, namely a knowledge of the degree of intoxication of the target population before adding a new source. In toxicology, the only absolute determinant that will dictate whether a toxic effect occurs is the body tissue concentration. Another worrying possibility is that these models can be run 'in reverse', starting with the answers required by the regulatory authorities, and arriving at an 'acceptable' solution by tinkering with the model until it fulfils the required endpoints. It is not known if this practice is widespread and it is almost impossible to find out. Nevertheless, in recognition of this possibility, risk assessment has been likened 'to a captured spy - if you torture it enough it will tell you anything you want to know'.

There is an urgent need to provide training for decision-makers in the evaluation of risk assessments, which can, on occasion, be little more than someone's opinion dressed up as a pseudo-scientific document.

In this respect, the proposal of the European Committee of Environmental Technology Suppliers Associations (EUCETSA) to establish a permanent discussion forum (Lindbauer, 2000) with representatives of industry sectors, authorities and NGOs, may be most useful, provided that all parties have an equal opportunity for input. On this platform the responsibility of the different social actors in a policy driven by precaution can be discussed and the principle can be acquainted.

## 5. Instruments to Make Waste Prevention Effective

Most instruments for environmental management react to pollution or other environmental damage. Only a limited number of them have proactive and preventive capacity (Hens, 1999). In the discussion on waste management three tools come to the forefront: health impact assessment, environmental taxes and environmental health education.

### *5.1. Health Impact Assessment*

In the US waste policy is to an important extent driven by risk analysis. In spite of major practical and methodological limitations (Johnston *et al.*, 1999), risk and the intimately linked hazard assessment are fundamental ingredients of health impact assessment (HIA). This methodology in its turn is an integral part of environmental impact assessment of projects (Hens, 2000). Moreover, as an SEA Directive is coming up, the EU is embarking on strategic environmental assessment of plans and programmes. In this context HIA should allow for the forecasting of health effects of different policy options and identify those with the least impact. The problem that the literature shows ample examples of the questionable use of risk assessment should be counteracted by paying increased attention to the quality control of both the statements and the process.

### *5.2. Environmental Taxes*

As industrial countries face growing amounts of household waste, moving away from landfill and incineration can only be realised by effective instruments to promote prevention of waste. Here Steenwegen's (2000) contribution on environmental taxes for selected waste streams, such as single-use bottles, might be most promising. Under well defined conditions such as clear targets, a motivated competent authority and an informed public, environmental taxes prove to be one of the few powerful instruments to prevent waste at its genesis.

### 5.3. *Environmental Education*

Moving environmental health issues to the centre of decision-making on waste policy necessitates the involvement of a wide array of target groups: health researchers, medical doctors, environmental professionals, decision-makers, science communicators, lawyers, insurance experts, industrial sectors, environmental and consumer NGOs and the public in general.

These different groups need to be properly informed about pollutants, their environmental fate, their effects, the evaluation of the effects, possible policy options and their consequences both in practical and ethical terms.

Because of this variety of subjects and the different target groups, an interdisciplinary approach to communicating the core of the matter is the only possible strategy. Nonetheless, the complexity of the problem should not mean that too opaque a message should be communicated. An important part of the exercise concerns the synthesis of the multidisciplinary elements in an accessible and easily-comprehended message.

'Chemical hygiene' might become part of this. Chemical hygiene finds its counterpart in microbiological hygiene. Health educators have been using this notion for almost a century. It led to a reduction in infant mortality and an increase in the quality of life. It entails living in a clean household environment, and includes personal hygiene. Chemical hygiene broadens the notion of microbiological hygiene in a number of ways:

- from biological organisms to the overwhelming number of chemicals in the environment. These latter should be limited to numbers which are necessary in a societal context. Such an attitude might reduce the number of man-made chemicals in the environment by a factor ranging between 10 and 100;
- from the private and personal environment to larger scales (from local to global) which matter in environmental problems;
- from the individual level (e.g. changing from scented soap to simple soap) to a societal level (e.g. changing from complex mixtures of chemicals like texaphene to single compound products), involving the main actors of environmental management, including business and industry, small- and medium-sized companies,

farmers, unions, women, youth, authorities, environmental and consumer NGOs and the public at large.

Next to microbiological hygiene, a chemical hygiene attitude might substantially improve life both in quantitative and qualitative terms.

Putting chemical hygiene on the agenda and moving environmental health concerns into the centre of decision-making on waste management will necessitate targeted action. A most necessary prerequisite to this is the training and education of all involved target groups. In view of the nature of these groups, both formal and non-formal education actions will be necessary.

These elements are most central in the 'Declaration of Kos' (Box 3). This text emerged as a consensus document from discussion among the participants in the workshop of which this book contains the proceedings. They mirror the opinion of a non-mandated, motivated and broad sample of the groups to be addressed.

The declaration emphasises:

- the main functional systems in the human body threatened by pollution in general and by pollution caused by waste deposit sites and incinerators in particular;
- the need for training and education both in its formal and the non-formal aspects. Special attention is given to environmental health in primary schools. Training of medical students and environmental professionals is specifically addressed;
- the need for an interdisciplinary approach to understand environmental health problems in their context and to be able to assess suggested solutions;
- the adoption of a chemical hygiene attitude.

A tool to put the 'Declaration of Kos' into practice is the TREEE-health net (Box 4). This initiative emerged from a round table discussion organised at the University of Athens in 1994. Participants were from Greece, France, Germany, the UK, DG XI of the EU, UNICEF and WHO. The core idea is to provide and inculcate information on environmental health. To this end the TREEE-health net uses a variety of approaches, including long distance learning, life-long learning and training of trainers.

*Box 3.* Declaration of Kos on the need for education concerning environment and health.

Brought together at the International Hippocrates Foundation on the Greek island of Kos, in the Aegean Sea, the scientists collaborating in the European Aspis programme declare:

1. as the world population grows and as human activities due to technological developments have an increasing impact on the environment, observations indicate that environmental pollution, man-made chemicals and environmental factors in general are affecting human health to a significant degree;
2. as many different aspects of human health are affected by environmental factors, this environment must be complementary for healthy intra-uterine development and for the intact functioning of the immune, endocrine, respiratory and reproductive systems, together with the higher functions of the human brain;
3. as the incidence of cancer, autoimmune and degenerative diseases have increased, coupled with a rise in the prevalence of asthma and infertility in many parts of the world during the last decades, and as there are good reasons to believe that environmental factors are at least in part responsible for the observed increases;
4. as human well-being is affected in many places by environmental pollution;
5. as human health and well-being are intimately related to the health and quality of plants, animals and ecosystems;

that there is a need for a coherent effort to include the different aspects of the link between environment and human health and well-being into educational and teaching programmes. The approach used should emphasise interdisciplinarity, or even better, transdisciplinarity, awareness and prevention. It is well understood that free access to, and diffusion of information is a necessary prerequisite.

The link between environment and human health should, in particular, receive due attention throughout the already densely loaded medical curricula. These curricula should be refocused. The education of other professionals and the curricula preparing for important functions in government, industry and the judiciary should include sufficient emphasis on the importance of environmental pollution to human health and well-being. And as the general population should adopt chemical hygiene (avoiding exposure to reactive or hormone-like chemicals) as a means of protecting health in an industrialised world, proper attention should be paid to the link between the environment and human health in early basic education dispensed to the population in general.

A specific target within the project concerns the development of a database which combines scientific information on environmental health with environmental and policy data on the same subject. This is an essential tool to answer the broad scope of questions on environmental health the different target groups seeking for information might raise. The methodology is based on the combination of existing literature and laboratory data banks into a more complex, integrated information system. The front end of this information system to be developed will be based on a user-friendly philosophy, depending on the expertise of the user (e.g., policy-makers, journalists, experts, etc.)

requesting for information. This part of the project is managed by the Department of Informatics (Prof. Dr. S. Theoborides) of Athens' university.

The TREEE-health net as a whole will be hosted in a European Centre based on the Aegean Island of Kos (Greece). This is the place of birth of Hippocrates, who is not only considered to be the founding father of empirical medicine, but also the first doctor to be concerned about environmental impacts of health.

## 6. Conclusions

This book reviews the health impacts which might result from waste deposit sites and incineration. Although the environmental mechanisms and exposure pathways to pollutants emerging from these events are different, they all seem to influence cancer, congenital malformations, the genetic material, neurological and behavioural functions, the immunologic system, reproduction and the (sex and thyroid) hormone balance.

Waste policy aimed at reducing these effects, should put more emphasis on prevention and re-use. Therefore a more pronounced application of the precautionary principle seems unavoidable.

Health impact assessment, environmental taxes and environmental health education might prove to be the most effective instruments the decision-maker has to realise this policy.

The availability and accessibility of the relevant scientific evidence to different target groups should be actively promoted in this environmental education context. More than ever before this seems a prerequisite to answer the growing concerns of society about issues of health and environment.

*Box 4.* TRans-European Environmental Educational Health Network (TREEE-Health net).

**Background**

Environmental pollution is increasingly impinging upon every day clinical medicine as a cause of morbidity and mortality. Despite a number of initiatives at governmental and EC levels this situation does not appear to be improving and in certain respects is actually deteriorating. However, the level of training offered as part of the medical curriculum across Europe is perceived to be low and indeed is absent from the majority of courses.

There is an urgent requirement, therefore, to increase the knowledge base of the medical profession in Europe. A longer term objective which could be perceived to be of general benefit to the European Community would be to raise the general awareness of the whole population by introducing and increasing the content of environmental information throughout the European education system at all levels from primary to tertiary establishments. Realising that we are living in the age of the 'screen' (computer, television, movie) it is obvious that young people are left with the alienating feeling that participation in every day problems such as environmental issues is not acceptable. So they encounter the accumulation of problems as a natural procedure without considering the possibility of legal action. Computers should be used in education to spread information and the matter should be handled with care.

**Aims**

TREEE-Health net aims 'to introduce environmental issues into Europe's educational systems at all levels and to increase general awareness of the impact of pollution, smoking, drug abuse, alcohol and radiation on the health and welfare of the community'.

This should cover all aspects of human health, including quality of life, which are determined by physical, biological, social and psychological factors in the environment, and should particularly concentrate on the possible long-term effects of today's activities for future generations.

**Objectives**

The activities of TREEE-Health net should:

- be designed in such a way that they have a multiplying effect across the whole of Europe;
- contain programmes for training trainers to facilitate the rapid dissemination of knowledge;
- have a balanced co-operation between the member states of the EU;
- be designed by combining scientific knowledge with cultural events (ancient theatre, concerts and guided happenings in museums) in order to develop a new attitude towards educational processes and to avoid dull experiences;
- be multidisciplinary in approach through the incorporation of partners other than medical professionals (physicists, lawyers, journalists, environmentalists, etc.);
- have a defined long-term goal which is achieved in steps by defining a series of short- to medium-term tasks;
- have the aim of becoming part of the 'life-long learning' initiative within the EU;
- provide 'distance-learning' facilities;
- be a non-governmental, non-partisan, non-denominational, non-profit organisation;
- avoid radicalisation and politicisation by promulgating information that has been published only after a process of reputable peer review and via a system of internal review before being released.

## References

Biggeri, A., Barbone, F., Lagazio, C., Massimo, B., and Stanta, G. (1996) Air pollution and lung cancer in Trieste, Italy: spatial analysis of risk as a function of distance from sources, *Environmental Health Perspectives* **104 (7),** 750-754.

Bridges, J.W. (1992) Consideration of possible impact on human health – Vol. 1, Proof of Evidence, Document A13, submitted in evidence to the UK Department of the Environment Public Enquiry into an application for Planning Permission for a Refuse to Energy Plant in Belvedere, Bexley, Kent, UK.

Brundtland, G.H. (1999) The scientific underpinning of policy, *Science* **277**, 457.

Deml, E., Mangelsdorf, I., and Greim, H. (1996) Chlorinated dibenzodioxins and dibenzofurans in blood and human milk of non-occupationally exposed persons living in the vicinity of a municipal waste incinerator, *Chemosphere* **33 (10)**, 1941-1950.

Déportes, I., Benoit-Guyod, J.L., and Zmirou, D. (1995) Hazard to man and the environment posed by the use of urban waste compost: a review, *The Science of the Total Environment* **172**, 197-222.

Dolk, H., Vrijheid, M., Armstrong, B., Abramsky, L., Bianchi, F., Garne, E., Nelen, V., Robert, E., Scott, J.E.S., Stone D., and Tenconi, R. (1998) Risk of congenital anomalies near hazardous-waste landfill sites in Europe: the EUROHAZCON study, *The Lancet* **352**, 423-427.

Elliott, P., Shaddick, G., Kleinschmidt, I., Jolley, D., Walls, P., Beresford, J., and Grundy, C. (1996) Cancer incidence near municipal solid waste incinerators in Great Britain, *British Journal of Cancer* **73**, 702-710.

Fischer, G., Schwalbe, R., Moller, M., Ostrowski, R., Hollender, J., and Dott, W. (1998) Airborne molds and their metabolites at workplaces in composting plants, *Mycoses* **41 (Suppl. 1)**, 51-55.

Goldberg, M.S., Al-Homsi, N., Goulet, L., and Riberdy, H. (1995a) Incidence of cancer among persons living near a municipal solid waste landfill site in Montreal Quebec, *Archives of Environmental Health* **50 (6)**, 416-424.

Goldberg, M.S., Goulet, L., Riberdy, H., and Bonvalot, Y. (1995b) Low birthweight and preterm births among infants born to women living near a municipal solid waste landfill site in Montreal, Quebec, *Environmental Research* **69**, 37-50.

Goldberg, M.S., Siemiatyck, J., DeWar, R., Désy, M., and Riberdy, H. (1999) Risks of developing cancer relative to living near a municipal solid waste landfill site in Montreal, Quebec, *Archives of Environmental Health* **54** **(4)**, 291-296.

Hens, L. (1994) The Rio-conference and thereafter, in B. Nath, L. Hens, and D. Devuyst (eds) *Sustainable Development*, VUB-Press, Brussels, Belgium, pp. 81-109.

Hens, L. (1999) Instruments for environmental management: introduction, in B. Nath, L. Hens, P. Compton, and D. Devuyst (eds) *Environmental Management in Practice, Vol. 1*, Routledge, London and New York, pp. 65-68.

Hens, L. (2000) Health and environmental impact assessment, in P. Nicolopoulou-Stamati, L. Hens, and C.V. Howard (eds) *Health Impacts of Waste Management Policies*, Kluwer Academic Publishers, Dordrecht, the Netherlands, pp. 175-198.

Hertzman, C., Hayes, M., Singer, J., and Highland, J. (1987) Upper Ottawa Street landfill site health study, *Environmental Health Perspectives* **75**, 173-195.

Holm, S., and Harris, J. (1999) Precautionary principle stifles discovery, *Nature* **400**, 398.

Howard, C.V., and Saunders, P.T. (1999) Sensible precautions make good science, *Nature* **401**, 207.

Ivens, U.I., Ebbehøj, N., Poulsen, O.M., and Skov, T. (1997) Season, equipment and job function related to gastro-intestinal problems in waste collectors, *Occupational and Environmental Medicine* **54**, 861-867.

Johnston, P., Stringer, R., Santillo, D., and Howard, C.V. (1999) Hazard, exposure and ecological risk assessment, in B. Nath, L. Hens, P. Compton, and D. Devuyst (eds) *Environmental Management in Practice, Vol. 1*, Routledge, London and New York, pp. 169-187.

Klekowski, E., and Levin, D.E. (1979) Mutagens in a river heavily polluted with paper recycling wastes: results of field and laboratory mutagen assays, *Environmental Mutagenesis* **1**, 209-219.

Klemans, W., Vleminckx, C., Schriewer, L., Joris, I., Lijsen, N., Maes, A., Ottogali, M., Pays, A., Planard, C., Rigaux, G., Ros, Y., Vande Rivière, M., Vandenvelde, J., Verschaeve, L., Deplaen, P., and Lakhanisky, T. (1995) Cytogenetic biomonitoring of a population of children allegedly exposed to environmental pollutants. Phase 2: Results of a three-year longitudinal study, *Mutation Research* **342**, 147-156.

Kramer, M.N., Kurup, V.P., and Fink, J.N. (1989) Allergic Bronchopulmonary Aspergillosis from a contaminated dump site, *American Review of Respiratory Diseases* **140**, 1086-1088.

Kurttio, P., Pekkanen, J., Alfthan, G., Paunio, M., Jaakkola, J., and Heinonen, O.P. (1998) Increased mercury poisoning in inhabitants living in the vicinity of a hazardous waste incinerator: a 10 year follow-up, *Archives of Environmental Health* **53**, 129-137.

Lakhanisky, T., Bazzoni, D., Jadot, P., Joris, I., Laurent, C., Ottogali, M., Pays, A., Planard, C., Ros, Y., and Vleminckx (1993) Cytogenetic monitoring of a village population potentially exposed to a low level of environmental pollutants. Phase 1: SCE analysis, *Mutation Research* **319**, 317-323.

Laurent, C., Lakhanisky, T., Jadot, P., Joris, I., Ottogali, M., Planard, C., Bazzoni, D., Foidart, J.M., and Ros, Y. (1993) Increased sister chromatid exchange frequencies observed in a cohort of inhabitants of a village located at the boundary of an industrial dumping ground: Phase 1, *Cancer Epidemiology, Biomarkers and Prevention* **2**, 355-362.

Lindbauer, R. (2000) Waste-to-energy and waste management: Austrian and EU policy lines, in P. Nicolopoulou-Stamati, L. Hens, and C.V. Howard (eds) *Health Impacts of Waste Management Policies*, Kluwer Academic Publishers, Dordrecht, the Netherlands, pp. 89-106.

Linher, O. (2000) Waste management: an industrial point of view, in P. Nicolopoulou-Stamati, L. Hens, and C.V. Howard (eds) *Health Impacts of Waste Management Policies*, Kluwer Academic Publishers, Dordrecht, the Netherlands, pp. 57-62.

Ma, X.F., Babish, J.G., Scarlett, J.M., Gutenmann, W.H., and Lisk, D.J. (1992) Mutagens in urine sampled repetitively from municipal refuse incinerator workers and water treatment, *Journal of Toxicology and Environmental Health* **37**, 483-494.

Mallin, K. (1990) Investigation of a bladder cancer cluster in North-western Illinois, *American Journal of Epidemiology* **132 (1)**, S96-S106.

Marth, E., Sixl, W., Bencko, V., Medwed, M., Lapajne, S., Voncina, E., and Brumen, S. (1995) People of the garbage dumps of Cairo: a toxicological in vivo model? *Central European Journal of Public Health* **3**, 154-157.

Michelozzi, P., Fusco, D., Forastiere, F., Ancona, C., Dell'Orco, V., and Perucci, C.A. (1998) Small area study of mortality among people living near multiple sources of air pollution, *Occupational and Environmental Medicine* **55**, 611-615.

Pani, B., Laureni, U., Babudri, N., Collareta, A., Venturini, S., Ferri, R., Carrozzi, M., Burlini, F., and Monti-Bragadin, C. (1983) Mutagenicity test of extracts of airborne dust from the municipal incinerator of Trieste, *Environmental Mutagenesis* **5**, 23-32.

Passman, F.J. (1983) Recovery of Aspergillus fumigatus aerospora from municipal sewage sludge composting operations in the state of Maine, *Mycopathologia* **83**, 41-51.

Poulsen, O., Breum, N., Ebbehøj, N., Hansen, A., Ivens, U., van Lelieveld, D., Malmros, P., Matthiasen, L., Nielsen, B., Nielsen, E., Schiby, B., Skov, T., Stenbaek, E., and Wilkins, K. (1995) Sorting and recycling of domestic waste. Review of occupational health problems and their possible causes, *The Science of the Total Environment* **168**, 33-56.

Rapiti, E., Sperati, A., Fano, V., Dell'Orco, V., and Forastiere, F. (1997) Mortality among workers at municipal waste incinerators in Rome: a retrospective cohort study, *American Journal of Industrial Medicine* **31**, 659-661.

Rix, B.A., and Lynge, E. (1996) Industrial hygiene measurements in a new industry: the repulping and deinking of paper waste, *American Journal of Industrial Medicine* **30**, 142-147.

Ruskbrook, P. (2000) The challenge to achieve better landfills where only dumps are achieved now: an anthology, in P. Nicolopoulou-Stamati, L. Hens, and C.V. Howard (eds) *Health Impacts of Waste Management Policies*, Kluwer Academic Publishers, Dordrecht, the Netherlands, 41-56.

Shy, C.M., Degnan, D., Fox, D.L., Mukerjee, S., Hazucha, M.J., Boehlecke, B.A., Rothenbacher, D., Briggs, P.M., Devlin, R.B., Wallace, D.D., Stevens, R.K., and Bromberg, P.A. (1995) Do waste incinerators induce adverse respiratory effects? An air quality and epidemiological study of six communities, *Environmental Health Perspectives* **103**, 714-724.

Steenwegen, K. (2000) Can ecological taxes play a role in diminishing the health impacts of waste management?, in P. Nicolopoulou-Stamati, L. Hens, and C.V. Howard (eds) *Health Impacts of Waste Management Policies*, Kluwer Academic Publishers, Dordrecht, the Netherlands, 199-214.

ten Tusscher, G., Stam, G.A, and Koppe, J.G. (2000) A local increased incidence of orofacial clefts in Amsterdam: the result of open combustion of chemicals?, in P. Nicolopoulou-Stamati, L. Hens, and C.V. Howard (eds) *Health Impacts of Waste*

*Management Policies*, Kluwer Academic Publishers, Dordrecht, the Netherlands, pp. 225-238.

Thorn, J., Beijer, L., and Rylander, R. (1998) Airways inflammation and glucan exposure among household waste collectors, *American Journal of Industrial Medicine* **33**, 463-470.

Tovalin-Ahumada, H. (1998) Health status of the population in the vicinity of a waste recycling plant in Mexico, *Revista Panamericana de Salud Publica* **3** (**1**), 15-20.

Valaoras, G. (2000) Waste management policies in the United States of America, in P. Nicolopoulou-Stamati, L. Hens, and C.V. Howard (eds) *Health Impacts of Waste Management Policies*, Kluwer Academic Publishers, Dordrecht, the Netherlands, pp. 121-132.

Van Larebeke, N. (2000) Health effects of a household waste incinerator near Wilrijk (Belgium), in P. Nicolopoulou-Stamati, L. Hens, and C.V. Howard (eds) *Health Impacts of Waste Management Policies*, Kluwer Academic Publishers, Dordrecht, the Netherlands, pp. 239-250.

Vardaka-Sotiropoulos, D. (2000) The European Environmental Bureau on the European Commission's Proposal on Incineration of Waste, in P. Nicolopoulou-Stamati, L. Hens, and C.V. Howard (eds) *Health Impacts of Waste Management Policies*, Kluwer Academic Publishers, Dordrecht, the Netherlands, pp. 65-72.

Williams, F.L.R., Lawson, A.B., and Lloyd, O.L. (1992) Low sex ratios of births in areas at risk from air pollution from incinerators, as shown by geographical analysis and 3-dimensional mapping, *International Journal of Epidemiology* **21** (**2**), 311-319.

Wrbitzky, R., Göen, T., Letzel, S., and Frank, F. (1995) Internal exposure of waste incineration workers to organic and inorganic substances, *International Archives of Occupational and Environmental Health* **68**, 13-21.

Zmirou, D., Parent, B., and Potelon, J-L. (1984) Etude épidémiologique des effets sur la santé des rejets atmosphériques d'une usine d'incinération de déchets industriels et ménagers, *Rev. Epidém. et Santé Publ.* **32**, 391-397. (in French)

# LIST OF ABBREVIATIONS

| | |
|---|---|
| AhR | Aryl hydrocarbon Receptor |
| AQO | Ambient Quality Objective |
| ASPIS | Awareness Strategies for Pollution from Industries |
| BAT | Best Available Technology |
| BATNEEC | Best Available Technology not Entailing Excessive Cost |
| BEP | Best Environmental Practice |
| BMA | British Medical Association |
| CBA | Cost-Benefit Analysis |
| CFC | Chloro-Fluoro-Carbon |
| DAV | Daily Average Value |
| DDT | Dichlor-Diphenyl-Trichlorethane |
| DETR | Department of the Environment, Transport and the Regions (UK) |
| DG | Directorate General |
| EAL | Environmental Assessment Level |
| EC | European Commission |
| EEB | European Environmental Bureau |
| EHIA | Environmental Health Impact Assessment |
| EIA | Environmental Impact Assessment |
| EIS | Environmental Impact Statement |
| ELV | Emission Limit Value |
| EPA | Environmental Protection Agency |
| EU | European Union |
| HAAV | Half-hourly Average Value |
| HCB | Hexachlorobenzene |
| HDN | Haemorrhagic Disease of the Newborn |
| HDPE | High Density Polyethylene |
| HIA | Health Impact Assessment |
| HREM | High Resolution Electron Microscope |
| IARC | International Association for Research on Cancer |
| IPC | Integrated Pollution Control |
| IPPC | Integrated Pollution Prevention and Control |
| IQ | Intelligence Quotient |
| I-TEQ | International Toxicity Equivalent |
| LBS | Land-Based Sources of Pollution |

| | |
|---|---|
| LCA | Life Cycle Analysis |
| LCP | Life Cycle Paralysis |
| $LD_{50}$ | Lethal Dose to 50 per cent of Animals |
| LDC | Less Developed Country |
| LPG | Liquid Petrol Gas |
| MAFF | Ministry of Agriculture, Farming and Fishery |
| MAP | Mediterranean Action Plan |
| MSW | Municipal Solid Waste |
| MWI | Municipal Waste Incinerator |
| NGO | Non-Governmental Organisation |
| NOAEL | No Observed Adverse Effect Level |
| NOEL | No Effect Level |
| NRC | National Research Council |
| OECD | Organisation of Economic Co-operation and Development |
| OVAM | Flemish Public Waste Agency |
| PBB | Polybrominated Biphenyls |
| PBDE | Polybrominated Diphenyl Ethers |
| PCB | Poly Chlorinated Biphenyl |
| PCDD | Polychlorinated Dibenzodioxins |
| PCDF | Polychlorinated Dibenzofurans |
| PM | Particulate Matter |
| POP | Persistent Organic Pollutant |
| PVA | Polyvinyl Alcohol |
| PVC | Polyvinyl Chloride |
| PxDF/D | Polybrominated and Mixed Dibenzofurans/dioxins |
| REHW | Rachel's Environment and Health Weekly |
| REIA | Regulatory and Environmental Impact Assessment |
| RfD | Reference Dose |
| SAP | Strategic Action Programme |
| SEA | Strategic Environmental Assessment |
| SELCHP | South East London Combined Heat and Power |
| SHW | Small Scale Hazardous Waste |
| TBT | Tributyltin |
| TCDD | 2,3,7,8-Tetrachlorodibenzo-p-dioxin |
| TDI | Tolerable Daily Intake |
| TEQ | Toxic Equivalence |
| TOC | Total Organic Carbon |
| ToR | Terms of Reference |
| TPB | Toxic, Persistent and Liable to Bio-accumulate Pollutant |
| TRH | Thyreotropic Releasing Hormone |
| TSH | Thyroid Stimulating Hormone |
| TSP | Total Suspended Particulate |
| UK | United Kingdom |
| UN | United Nations |
| US(A) | United States (of America) |
| US EPA | United States Environmental Protection Agency |

| | |
|---|---|
| VFG-waste | Vegetable, Fruit and Garden Waste |
| W/W | Weight to Weight |
| WHO | World Health Organisation |
| WHO-TEQ | WHO Toxicity Equivalents |

# LIST OF UNITS

## Prefixes to Units

| | | | | | |
|---|---|---|---|---|---|
| da | deca | $(10^{1})$ | d | deci | $(10^{-1})$ |
| h | hecto | $(10^{2})$ | c | centi | $(10^{-2})$ |
| k | kilo | $(10^{3})$ | m | milli | $(10^{-3})$ |
| M | Mega | $(10^{6})$ | µ | micro | $(10^{-6})$ |
| G | Giga | $(10^{9})$ | n | nano | $(10^{-9})$ |
| T | Tera | $(10^{12})$ | p | pico | $(10^{-12})$ |
| P | Peta | $(10^{15})$ | f | femto | $(10^{-15})$ |

## Units

| | | | |
|---|---|---|---|
| BF | Belgian Frank | $Nm^3$ | Normalised cubic metre |
| °C | degree Celcius or centigrade | pa | per annum |
| d | day | pH | acidity |
| Drachmas | Greek currency unit | ppb | parts per billion |
| Euro | European currency unit | ppm | parts per million |
| g | gram | s | second |
| h | hour | t | ton |
| $kg_{bw}$ | kilogram body weight | te | ton emission gas |
| kgpa | kilogram per annum | tpa | ton per annum |
| l | litre | US$ | US Dollar |
| m | metre | y | year |

# INDEX